THE CASTOR OIL HANDBOOK

Your Complete Guide to Unleashing the Natural Benefits for Health, Beauty, DIY Recipes and FAQ

Dr Bailey Castro

Disclaimer

The information contained in this book is for educational and informational purposes only and is not intended as health or medical advice. The author and publisher are not responsible for any specific health or allergy needs that may require medical supervision and are not liable for any damages or negative consequences from any treatment, action, application, or preparation to any person reading or following the information in this book. References are provided for informational purposes only and do not constitute an endorsement of any websites or other sources.

TABLE OF CONTENTS

Chapter One

Introduction to Castor Oil

When children showed the first signs of illness, many parents and grandparents would quickly give castor oil to their children, either topically or internally, in order to naturally improve immune function and speed up the healing process. Since the beginning of time, this activity has been carried out.

Over the course of thousands of years, it has also been utilized by traditional healers all over the world to treat a wide range of health ailments. Castor oil, for instance, has been used by ancient Egyptians to treat eye irritations and as a potent natural skin care remedy. This practice dates back to the time when castor oil was considered among the most beneficial substances.

Ayurvedic medicine makes use of it since it is believed to be an antibacterial, skin-healing, and digestive-soothing element. It also has deep origins in India, where it is considered to be healing to the skin.

What is the current application of castor oil? As is further discussed in this book, it possesses naturally stimulating laxative characteristics; it has been demonstrated to improve lymphatic, circulatory, and immunological health; and it can assist in the treatment of a variety of conditions, including arthritis, constipation, and others.

What is Castor Oil?

Castor oil is a type of vegetable oil that has been utilized for a significant amount of time due to the numerous therapeutic and medicinal activities that it possesses. The Ricinus communis plant, which is indigenous to tropical regions of Africa and India but is now cultivated in many parts of the world, is the source of this substance. It is acquired from the seeds of this plant. Because of its diverse composition and extensive range of applications in the fields of health, beauty, and industry, the oil that is derived from these seeds is highly regarded.

Physical Characteristics

Castor oil is a pale yellow, viscous liquid with a modest, identifiable odor and a somewhat nutty taste. It is characterized by its high viscosity and density, making it thicker than many other vegetable oils. These unique physical features contribute to its success in different applications, particularly in its capacity to coat and protect surfaces, such as skin and hair.

History and Origins

Ancient Beginnings

Castor oil has a long history of use dating back to prehistoric times, with records indicating its existence in various early cultures. The Egyptians were among the first to recognize and make use of the benefits of castor oil; castor seeds have been found in Egyptian tombs dating back to 4000 BCE, and the oil was frequently used in lamps, cosmetics, and medicinal purposes. In addition to using it as a laxative (a practice that is still practiced in some societies today), Egyptians applied castor oil to their skin to protect it from the harsh desert environment and to promote wound healing.

In ancient Greece and Rome, castor oil was similarly esteemed. Greek physicians such as Hippocrates and Dioscorides noted its medical benefits, mainly for stomach disorders and as a poultice for skin ailments. The oil was also utilized in the manufacture of balms and ointments.

Castor Oil in Ayurvedic Medicine

In India, castor oil has a long history of usage in Ayurvedic medicine, a holistic healing method that has been practiced for over 3,000 years. Ayurvedic practitioners employed castor oil for its purgative effects, as well as for treating inflammatory diseases and skin ailments. The oil was believed to balance the body's doshas (vital energies) and was commonly used in massage therapy and other healing rites.

Spread and Adoption

As trade channels increased, the usage of castor oil spread to various parts of the world. In the Middle Ages, castor oil was introduced to Europe, where it became a popular cure for different diseases. By the 18th and 19th centuries, castor oil was widely used in Europe and North America, largely as a laxative and for treating skin disorders.

Modern Era

In the 20th century, the industrial applications of castor oil began to be studied. The oil's peculiar chemical qualities make it acceptable for use in the creation of soaps, lubricants, hydraulic fluids, and even as a component in polymers and synthetic resins. During World War I and World War II, castor oil was employed as a lubricant for aircraft engines due to its high lubricity and stability at low temperatures.

Today, castor oil remains a versatile and valuable resource, with continuous use in traditional medicine, modern pharmaceuticals, cosmetics, and many industrial applications.

Understanding its Composition

Chemical Structure

Ricinoleic acid, which is a monounsaturated omega-9 fatty acid, is the primary component of castor oil.

Ricinoleic acid makes up nearly 90% of the fatty acid content in castor oil, giving it specific qualities that separate it from other vegetable oils. The chemical structure of ricinoleic acid includes a hydroxyl group, which contributes to the oil's high viscosity and solubility in alcohol, as well as its antibacterial and anti-inflammatory characteristics.

Fatty Acid Profile

In addition to ricinoleic acid, castor oil includes numerous additional fatty acids, including:

Oleic Acid (6%): A monounsaturated omega-9 fatty acid recognized for its moisturizing and anti-inflammatory qualities.

Linoleic Acid (4%): A polyunsaturated omega-6 fatty acid that plays a critical function in preserving skin health and integrity.

Palmitic Acid (1%): A saturated fatty acid that serves to stabilize the oil and extend its shelf life.

Stearic Acid (1%): A saturated fatty acid that contributes to the oil's thick, rich texture.

This particular fatty acid makeup makes castor oil very emollient, offering deep hydration and nourishment to the skin and hair.

Other Compounds

In addition to its fatty acids, castor oil includes several additional substances that increase its medicinal qualities. These include:

Vitamin E: An antioxidant that helps protect the skin from damage caused by free radicals and environmental stresses.

Minerals: Trace minerals that enhance general skin health and function.

Phytochemicals: Plant-based substances with anti-inflammatory, antibacterial, and therapeutic capabilities.

Extraction Process of Castor Oil

When it comes to extracting castor oil from castor seeds, the process is quite complicated and involves a number of different processes in order to obtain the highest possible quality oil. In order to provide a comprehensive overview of the complete procedure:

1. Harvesting

Materials Involved: Mature castor bean plants (Ricinus communis).

Process: Castor seeds are gathered from the plant when they are fully grown, which is often indicated by the drying and cracking of the seed pods. Mature seeds contain the maximum proportion of oil.

2. Cleaning and Drying

Materials Involved: Castor seeds, cleaning equipment (e.g., air blowers, sieves).

Process: The gathered seeds are washed to eliminate dirt, debris, and other contaminants. This is commonly done using air blowers, sieves, or similar equipment. After cleaning, the seeds are dried to minimize their moisture content, which aids in the extraction process and prevents spoiling. Both sun-drying techniques and mechanical dryers can be used for drying.

3. Extraction

One of the two primary techniques for extracting castor oil is expeller pressing or cold pressing.

Cold Pressing

Materials Involved: Castor seeds, cold press machine.

Process:

Preparation: The cleaned and dried seeds are placed into a cold press machine.

Mechanism: The seeds are mechanically pressed without the application of heat. This process entails employing a screw press that crushes the seeds and expels the oil.

Benefits: Cold pressing protects the oil's natural nutrients, antioxidants, and beneficial components, leading to a higher quality and more nutrient-rich oil. Cold-pressed castor oil is frequently more expensive due to its labor-intensive method and lesser yield.

Yield: Lower compared to expeller pressing, but the oil keeps more of its natural qualities.

Expeller Pressing

Materials Involved: Castor seeds, expeller press machine.

Process:

Preparation: The cleaned and dried seeds are placed into an expeller press machine.

Mechanism: The seeds are exposed to mechanical pressure mixed with heat created by friction. The heat helps to extract more oil from the seeds.

Benefits: Expeller pressing generates a larger yield of oil compared to cold pressing, making it a more cost-effective approach. However, the application of heat can damage some of the oil's beneficial properties, leading to a lesser quality oil in terms of purity and nutrient content.

Yield: Higher than cold pressing, but may include less useful chemicals.

4. Filtration and Refining

Materials Involved: Filter equipment, refining agents (if necessary).

Process:

Filtration: The crude oil recovered from either technique is filtered to eliminate solid contaminants such as seed remnants, debris, and other particles. Filtration can be done using many ways such as mechanical filters, centrifuges, or textile filters.

Refining: The filtered oil may undergo additional refining operations to increase its quality, including neutralization, decolorization, and deodorization. This procedure guarantees that the oil is free from contaminants and has a suitable color and odor. Refined oil is frequently more consistent in quality and appearance.

Materials Involved:

Cold Press Machine: Used for cold pressing to protect oil's natural qualities.

Expeller Press Machine: Used for expeller pressing to obtain a bigger volume of oil.

Filtering Equipment: Includes mechanical filters, centrifuges, and textile filters for eliminating contaminants.

Refining Agents: Chemicals and agents used throughout the refining process to enhance the oil's purity.

This extensive extraction procedure guarantees that castor oil is obtained in its most useable form, with the choice of method determining the oil's final quality and cost

Modern Applications of Castor Oil

Castor oil offers a varied variety of current applications due to its unique qualities and benefits. Here's a detailed look at how castor oil is used in several fields today:

1. Personal Care and Beauty

a. Skincare

Hydration: Castor oil is known for its profound hydrating effects. It is often used in skincare products such as lotions, creams, and serums to give moisture and enhance skin suppleness.

Anti-Aging: Rich in antioxidants, castor oil helps counteract free radicals, which can contribute to skin aging. It is used in anti-aging lotions and serums to minimize the appearance of fine lines and wrinkles.

Acne Treatment: The oil's antibacterial and anti-inflammatory characteristics make it beneficial in treating acne and lowering inflammation and redness associated with outbreaks.

b. Hair Care

Hair Growth: Castor oil is known for its role in encouraging hair growth. It is used in shampoos, conditioners, and hair masks to improve scalp health, strengthen hair follicles, and minimize hair loss.

Conditioning: The oil functions as a deep conditioner, making hair smoother and more manageable. It provides gloss and aids in keeping moisture in.

c. Nail and Cuticle Care

Strengthening Nails: Castor oil is used in nail care products to strengthen nails, eliminate brittleness, and promote healthy nail growth.

Moisturizing Cuticles: It is also used to cuticles to keep them hydrated, reducing dryness and cracking.

2. Medical and Therapeutic Uses

a. Pain Relief

Joint Pain: Castor oil's anti-inflammatory qualities make it effective for alleviating joint pain and arthritis symptoms. It is typically used in warm compresses or administered topically to afflicted regions.

Muscle Soreness: Used in massages, castor oil helps relax muscles and ease soreness.

b. Digestive Health

Constipation Relief: Castor oil is traditionally used as a laxative to ease constipation. It works by promoting bowel movements.

Digestive Health: The oil's ability to promote digestion and detoxify the liver makes it a popular choice for boosting digestive health.

c. Wound Healing

Minor Wounds and Infections: Castor oil is used in wound care to improve healing and prevent infection due to its antibacterial qualities. It can be administered topically to small wounds and abrasions.

3. Household Uses

a. Lubrication

Mechanical Lubricant: Castor oil's high viscosity makes it an effective lubricant for machinery and equipment, decreasing friction and wear.

b. Cleaning

Natural Cleaner: The oil is utilized in homemade cleaning products for its ability to break down grease and grime. It can be used in recipes for natural cleaning solutions.

4. Industrial Applications

a. Manufacturing

Industrial Lubricants: Castor oil is utilized in the creation of industrial lubricants due to its outstanding lubricating qualities and ability to tolerate high temperatures.

Plasticizers: To increase flexibility and durability in plastics, castor oil is utilized as a plasticizer throughout the production process.

b. Cosmetics and Pharmaceuticals

Cosmetic Formulations: Castor oil is a common ingredient in cosmetics, including lipsticks, lip glosses, and moisturizers, due to its emollient characteristics.

Pharmaceuticals: It is used in the manufacturing of some pharmaceuticals, including those for digestive health and skin treatments.

5. Alternative Therapies

a. Aromatherapy

Carrier Oil: Castor oil is used as a carrier oil in aromatherapy to dilute essential oils. It helps to distribute the essential oils to the skin and increases their absorption.

b. Detoxification

Castor Oil Packs: Used in alternative medicine, castor oil packs are applied to the belly or other locations to stimulate detoxification and maintain liver function.

Benefits Across Applications

Versatility: Castor oil's extensive range of applications indicates its versatility and adaptability in numerous sectors.

Natural and Effective: As a natural product, castor oil is valued for its effectiveness and has few adverse effects compared to synthetic alternatives.

Sustainability: Castor oil is obtained from the seeds of the castor bean plant, making it a sustainable solution for many uses.

Castor oil's modern applications stretch across personal care, medical treatments, industrial usage, and alternative therapies, highlighting its vital significance in contemporary health and wellness practices.

Chapter Two

The Benefits of Castor Oil

Health Benefits

Castor oil has been acclaimed for its various health advantages, mainly mostly to its unique chemical composition. The high quantity of ricinoleic acid, together with other therapeutic ingredients, makes castor oil a flexible and potent natural treatment. Below are specific insights into its health advantages, concentrating on immune system boosting and its pain relief and anti-inflammatory qualities.

Immune System Boost

Castor oil is believed to have immunostimulatory effects, which can assist in strengthening the body's natural defense mechanisms. This is partly due to its ability to increase lymphatic circulation and promote cleansing.

Lymphatic System Support

The lymphatic system plays a critical part in the body's immune response by delivering lymph, a fluid containing white blood cells that fight infections. When the lymphatic system is operating efficiently, it helps eliminate toxins, waste, and other undesired items from the body. It has been shown that castor oil enhances lymphatic function, which boosts immunity.

Application: Castor oil packs, where a cloth soaked in castor oil is placed on the skin (typically over the belly) and covered with heat, have been used to activate the lymphatic system. This technique can promote lymphatic circulation and improve general immune function.

Case Study: Lymphatic Congestion

Jane, a 45-year-old woman, has been enduring frequent infections and colds. She was often weary and thought her immune system was not operating properly. After consulting with a natural health practitioner, she started using castor oil packs. Jane put the pack on her abdomen three times a week. After a few weeks, she observed a considerable increase in her energy levels and a decrease in the frequency of her infections. Her practitioner attributed these advantages to the increased lymphatic circulation promoted by the castor oil packs.

Detoxification

Castor oil assists in the detoxification process, which is necessary for maintaining a healthy immune system. By boosting the body's ability to expel pollutants, castor oil can lower the stress on the immune system, allowing it to work more efficiently.

Application: Regular usage of castor oil packs can enhance liver function, aiding in the detoxification process. This can be particularly advantageous for persons exposed to high amounts of environmental pollutants or those with a history of poor food habits.

Case Study: Detoxification

In the case of Mark, a 50-year-old male, has a history of heavy alcohol intake and a diet high in processed foods. He constantly encountered intestinal troubles and thought his entire health was failing. His naturopath recommended including castor oil packs into his detox routine. After a month of constant use, Mark noted improved digestion, better skin color, and a sense of overall well-being. His liver function tests also showed improvement, showing the usefulness of the castor oil in assisting his detoxification process.

Pain Relief and Anti-Inflammatory Properties

One of the most well-known benefits of castor oil is its ability to ease pain and reduce inflammation. The high concentration of ricinoleic acid in castor oil is principally responsible for these effects.

Anti-Inflammatory Properties

Ricinoleic acid has been demonstrated to have powerful anti-inflammatory effects. It works by preventing the development of specific pro-inflammatory chemicals, ultimately lowering inflammation in the body.

Application: Topical application of castor oil to inflamed areas can provide relief from ailments such as arthritis, muscle soreness, and joint pain. Massaging the oil into the skin might help reduce swelling and improve healing.

Case Study: Arthritis Relief

Sarah, a 60-year-old lady with rheumatoid arthritis, endured continuous pain and stiffness in her joints. She was seeking a natural solution to supplement her conventional therapy. After learning about the anti-inflammatory properties of castor oil, Sarah began rubbing the oil into her damaged joints every day. Within a few weeks, she observed a considerable reduction in discomfort and an improvement in her joint mobility. Sarah continued to use castor oil as part of her arthritis management plan, finding it to be a helpful addition to her treatment program.

Pain Relief

Castor oil's analgesic qualities can give efficient pain relief for numerous diseases. It is particularly beneficial for reducing pain linked with muscle soreness, back discomfort, and menstrual cramps.

Application: For muscle tightness and back pain, massage castor oil into the affected area can bring relief. For menstrual cramps, placing a warm castor oil pack on the lower belly can help ease pain.

Case Study: Menstrual Cramp Relief

Emily, a 25-year-old woman, suffered from severe menstrual pains that often left her bedridden. Seeking a natural treatment, she tried using castor oil packs during her monthly period. She put the pack on her lower belly for 30 minutes each day during her period. Emily discovered that the castor oil substantially alleviated her cramps and allowed her to carry on with her usual activities. She was happy to have found a natural and efficient answer for her monthly pain.

Case Study: Back Pain Relief

John, a 40-year-old guy, has chronic lower back pain due to his sedentary profession. Traditional medicines provided temporary relief, but he was looking for a more durable alternative. John started applying castor oil to his lower back and observed a dramatic reduction in pain following regular application. He combined the castor oil application with modest stretching exercises, which significantly improved his condition. John's back pain became more manageable, allowing him to focus better on his work and daily activities.

Digestive Health

Castor oil has long been renowned for its strong effects on digestive health. Its most notable usage in this area is as a natural laxative, but it also possesses other qualities that can aid in keeping a healthy digestive tract.

Natural Laxative

The principal usage of castor oil for digestive health is as a stimulant laxative. Ricinoleic acid, the major component of castor oil, attaches to receptors on the smooth muscle cells of the intestinal wall, forcing those muscles to contract and push feces through the intestines.

Application: For relief from constipation, a small amount of castor oil (usually 1-2 teaspoons for adults) can be given orally. It normally takes action within 2-6 hours, therefore it's advisable to take it when you can remain at home.

Case Study: Relief from Constipation

Maria, a 30-year-old lady, frequently experienced constipation due to her busy lifestyle and irregular eating habits. After battling with over-the-counter laxatives that often produced discomfort, Maria decided to try castor oil. She took one tablespoon of castor oil in the evening, and by the next morning, she had great relief without the extreme cramping she had with previous treatments. Maria now takes castor oil as her go-to cure for periodic constipation, appreciating its natural efficiency.

Gut Health

Castor oil's anti-inflammatory effects can also aid gut health. By lowering inflammation in the intestines, it can help ease symptoms of numerous digestive illnesses.

Application: Castor oil packs applied to the abdomen can help reduce inflammation and enhance overall digestive health. This approach is very effective for patients with inflammatory bowel diseases like IBS (Irritable Bowel Syndrome).

Case Study: Managing IBS Symptoms

David, a 35-year-old man with IBS, experienced recurrent abdominal pain and bloating. Traditional drugs provided little help, so he investigated alternative therapy. David started applying castor oil packs on his belly three times a week. After a month of constant use, he saw a considerable reduction in his symptoms, including less discomfort and bloating. Castor oil packs became a vital element of David's IBS management approach, considerably enhancing his quality of life.

Beauty Benefits

Castor oil is a multipurpose cosmetic treatment, that has multiple advantages for skin, hair, and nails. Its rich, emollient characteristics make it an ideal addition to any beauty routine.

Skin Care

Castor oil is particularly good for the skin due to its hydrating, anti-inflammatory, and antibacterial characteristics. It can be used to treat a range of skin disorders and enhance overall skin health.

Moisturizing

Castor oil is an excellent moisturizer, capable of entering deeply into the skin to hydrate and nourish.

Application: A small amount of castor oil can be applied to the face and body as a natural moisturizer. It is especially beneficial for skin that is sensitive or dry.

Case Study: Winter Skin Relief

Anna, a 28-year-old lady, suffers from severely dry skin during the winter months. She realized that normal lotions were not giving adequate moisture. Anna started using castor oil on her skin before bed, focusing on particularly dry areas like her elbows and knees. Within a week, she observed a substantial change in her skin's moisture and texture. Castor oil became her go-to solution for treating winter dryness.

Treating Acne

Castor oil's antibacterial characteristics make it beneficial in treating acne and decreasing outbreaks.

Application: To treat acne, castor oil can be used directly on blemishes or used as part of an oil-washing program. Its anti-inflammatory effects can also help reduce redness and swelling associated with acne.

Case Study: Acne Management

Michael, a 20-year-old college student, had been dealing with acne for years. Traditional acne treatments typically left his skin dry and inflamed. He started using castor oil as part of his nightly beauty routine, massaging it into his face and then removing it with a warm cloth. After a few weeks, Michael observed fewer breakouts and an overall improvement in his skin's appearance. Castor oil helped him obtain brighter, healthier skin without the harsh side effects of standard therapies.

Healing Wounds and Scars

Castor oil enhances wound healing and minimizes the appearance of scars due to its capacity to encourage tissue growth.

Application: Applying castor oil to minor cuts, wounds, and scars can help speed up the healing process and enhance the appearance of scars over time.

Case Study: Scar Reduction

Lucy, a 35-year-old lady, had a prominent scar on her forearm from a previous incident. After reading about the healing effects of castor oil, she decided to apply it to her scar every day. Over several months, Lucy noted a progressive shrinking of the scar and an improvement in the texture of the skin. She was happy with the outcomes and continues to use castor oil for additional minor skin ailments.

Hair Care

Castor oil is commonly used in hair care for its ability to nourish the scalp, encourage hair growth, and improve hair texture.

Promoting Hair Growth

Castor oil is claimed to encourage hair growth by improving blood circulation to the scalp and giving necessary nutrients.

Application: To promote hair development, castor oil can be massaged into the scalp and left on for a few hours or overnight before rinsing it off. Mixing it with other oils like coconut or olive oil might make it simpler to apply and rinse out.

Case Study: Hair Growth

Jennifer, a 40-year-old lady, noticed receding hair after motherhood. She began using a mixture of castor oil and coconut oil on her scalp twice a week, leaving it on overnight. After three months, Jennifer saw fresh hair growth and general improvement in the thickness and condition of her hair. Castor oil became a fixture in her hair care routine, helping her recover confidence in her looks.

Conditioning and Strengthening Hair

Castor oil's rich, emollient characteristics help maintain and strengthen hair, making it smoother and less prone to breakage.

Application: For a thorough conditioning treatment, castor oil can be applied to the hair, from roots to ends, and left on for a few hours before washing it out.

Case Study: Deep Conditioning

Tom, a 30-year-old guy, has dry, brittle hair due to regular styling and exposure to harsh weather. He started using castor oil as a weekly deep conditioning treatment. After a few weeks, Tom observed his hair was substantially softer, shinier, and more robust. Castor oil helped restore moisture and strength to his hair, making it easier to handle.

Treating Scalp Conditions

Castor oil's antibacterial and anti-inflammatory characteristics make it beneficial in treating different scalp disorders, such as dandruff and itching.

Application: Applying castor oil massages to the scalp might help relieve inflamed scalps and minimize dandruff. Before washing it off, you can leave it on for a few hours or overnight.

Case Study: Dandruff Relief

Emma, a 25-year-old lady, struggled with dandruff and an itchy scalp. She began applying castor oil to her scalp once a week, putting it on overnight. After a month, Emma noted a dramatic reduction in dandruff and itching. Her scalp felt better, and her hair looked shinier and more vivid. Castor oil gave a natural and effective treatment for her scalp troubles.

Nail and Cuticle Care

Castor oil is beneficial for keeping healthy nails and cuticles due to its hydrating and strengthening characteristics.

Moisturizing Cuticles

Infections and painful hangnails can result from dry cuticles. Cuticles can remain healthy and hydrated with the use of castor oil.

Application: A small amount of castor oil can be massaged into the cuticles regularly to maintain them hydrated and prevent dryness.

Case Study: Healthy Cuticles

Sophia, a 35-year-old lady, often experienced dry, cracked cuticles, especially during the winter. She started applying castor oil on her cuticles every night before bed. After a few weeks, Sophia noted her cuticles were much smoother and healthier, and she no longer had unpleasant hangnails. Castor oil became a significant element of her nighttime routine for maintaining lovely hands.

Strengthening Nails

Brittle, weak nails might benefit from the nourishing characteristics of castor oil, which helps strengthen and protect them.

Application: Regular application of castor oil to the nails might help strengthen them and prevent breaking. Massaging the oil into the nails and surrounding skin helps enhance overall nail health.

Case Study: Nail Strengthening

Rachel, a 28-year-old woman, had weak, brittle nails that often broke and split. She began massaging castor oil into her nails and cuticles every evening. After a few months, Rachel found that her nails were stronger and less prone to breaking. The castor oil therapy altered her nails, making them healthier and more robust.

Castor oil is a great natural medicine with a wide range of benefits for digestive health and appearance. Its efficiency as a natural laxative and its capacity to improve gut health make it a vital supplement to any digestive health regimen. In the world of beauty, castor oil's hydrating, anti-inflammatory, and antibacterial characteristics give substantial advantages for the skin, hair, and nails. Whether you want to improve digestive function, enhance your skincare routine, encourage hair development, or maintain healthy nails and cuticles, castor oil offers a diverse and natural option. Through several case studies, the efficacy of castor oil in diverse uses is clearly established, showcasing its enduring importance in both traditional and modern health and beauty

Chapter Three

Choosing the Right Castor Oil

When it comes to selecting the appropriate castor oil, understanding the many varieties available and what to look for will help you make an informed decision. This article will discuss the numerous varieties of castor oil, the distinctions between cold-pressed and expeller-pressed oils, the benefits of organic vs. non-organic alternatives, how to read labels and certifications, and where to buy high-quality castor oil.

Types of Castor Oil

Castor oil comes in numerous kinds, each with its particular qualities and purposes. The primary varieties of castor oil include:

Cold-Pressed Castor Oil: Extracted without using heat, maintaining more nutrients and beneficial components.

Expeller-Pressed Castor Oil: Uses heat and pressure during extraction, which can destroy some nutrients but normally results in a larger yield.

Hydrogenated Castor Oil (Castor Wax): Created by adding hydrogen to castor oil, rendering it solid at room temperature; extensively used in cosmetics and industrial uses.

Jamaican Black Castor Oil: Made by roasting the castor seeds before pressing, resulting in a darker oil with a smokey fragrance; popular for hair treatment due to its purported hair growth benefits.

Organic Castor Oil: Certified organic, meaning it is free from synthetic pesticides and fertilizers.

Each variety has its specific uses, and the choice relies on your personal needs.

Cold-Pressed vs. Expeller-Pressed

Cold-Pressed Castor Oil

Extraction Process: Cold-pressed castor oil is obtained by pressing the castor seeds without adding heat. This process protects more of the oil's inherent nutrients and useful ingredients, such as vitamins, minerals, and fatty acids.

Nutritional Value: Cold-pressed castor oil is rich in ricinoleic acid, antioxidants, and other compounds that can be good for health and beauty purposes.

Price: Typically more expensive because of the lower yield and more labor-intensive extraction method.

Expeller-Pressed Castor Oil

Extraction Process: Expeller-pressed castor oil is created by pressing the seeds using heat and mechanical pressure. This approach results in a larger production of oil but can destroy some of the beneficial chemicals.

Nutritional Value: While expeller-pressed castor oil still contains ricinoleic acid and other minerals, it may have lesser quantities of some vitamins and antioxidants compared to cold-pressed oil.

Price: Generally, more affordable than cold-pressed oil due to the higher yield and less laborious extraction procedure.

Choosing Between Cold-Pressed and Expeller-Pressed

The decision between cold-pressed and expeller-pressed castor oil relies on your intended purpose. For skincare, hair care, and other personal applications where nutrient retention is vital, cold-pressed oil is ideal. For industrial usage or where budget is a factor, expeller-pressed oil may be a suitable option.

Organic vs. Non-Organic

Organic Castor Oil

Farming Practices: Castor beans grown without the use of artificial fertilizers, herbicides, or pesticides are the source of organic castor oil. This ensures that there are no hazardous chemical leftovers in the oil.

Certifications: Organic castor oil often has certificates from recognized authorities such as USDA Organic or ECOCERT, confirming conformity to organic production standards.

Environmental Impact: Organic farming practices are often more sustainable and environmentally benign, increasing soil health and biodiversity.

Non-Organic Castor Oil

Farming Practices: Non-organic castor oil is made from castor beans that may be farmed using synthetic chemicals. These procedures can leave residues in the oil and may have a bigger environmental impact.

Price: Non-organic castor oil is usually more affordable due to the reduced cost of conventional cultivation methods.

Quality: While non-organic castor oil can still be beneficial for many uses, it may not be as pure or environmentally benign as organic oil.

Choosing Between Organic and Non-Organic

For personal care and health uses, organic castor oil is typically the ideal choice due to its purity and lack of chemical residues. If cost is an important consideration or the oil is intended for non-personal usage, non-organic castor oil can be a suitable alternative.

Reading Labels and Certifications

When purchasing castor oil, it's crucial to study the labels and certifications to ensure you're obtaining a high-quality product. Here are a few essential components to look for:

Ingredients: The label should list 100% pure castor oil as the single ingredient. Avoid items with additional chemicals, perfumes, or fillers.

Certifications: Look for certificates such as USDA Organic, ECOCERT, or other recognized organic certification authorities. These certificates show that the oil satisfies particular organic criteria.

Extraction Method: The label should mention whether the oil is cold-pressed or expeller-pressed. Cold-pressed oil is ideal for most personal care uses.

Packaging: High-quality castor oil is often stored in dark glass bottles to protect it from light and oxidation, which can decrease the oil's quality over time.

Understanding Certifications

USDA Organic: Indicates that the oil is derived from castor beans grown according to USDA organic standards, without synthetic pesticides or fertilizers.

ECOCERT: A European certification that confirms the product fulfills specified organic and natural cosmetic criteria.

Non-GMO: Indicates that the castor beans used to create the oil are not genetically engineered.

Where to Buy High-Quality Castor Oil

You may purchase premium castor oil in a variety of locations, including physical and internet retailers. The following advice will help you find castor oil and know what to search for:

Health Food Stores

Availability: Health food stores generally have high-quality, organic castor oil. The team can also give advice depending on your individual needs.

Brands: Look for respected brands known for their quality and purity, such as Heritage Store, Now Solutions, and Sky Organics.

Online Retailers

Convenience: Online stores like Amazon, iHerb, and Vitacost offer a large assortment of castor oil products. Be cautious to read reviews and check for certifications to ensure quality.

Direct from Manufacturers: Purchasing directly from the manufacturer's website can verify authenticity and provide access to a greater variety of products.

Pharmacies

Availability: Many pharmacies have castor oil, often in the health and wellness section. While the choices may be limited, you can still discover decent products.

Brands: Look for well-known pharmacy brands that promote quality and safety.

Specialty Stores

Beauty and Wellbeing Shops: Specialty stores that focus on natural beauty and well-being items often stock high-quality castor oil. These stores often offer expert guidance and a chosen selection of products.

Farmers' Markets

Local Options: Farmers' markets may feature vendors offering locally sourced and produced castor oil. This option supports local companies and ensures a fresh, high-quality product.

Tips for Purchasing

Check Reviews: Reading customer reviews might provide insights into the quality and effectiveness of castor oil.

Compare costs: While price isn't usually an indicator of quality, exceptionally cheap costs can be a red flag for diluted or lower-quality oil.

Look for Dark Glass Bottles: High-quality castor oil is generally packaged in dark glass bottles to protect it from light and maintain its integrity.

Chapter four

Using Castor Oil for Health

Castor oil is recognized for its health advantages and various applications. It can be used both internally and externally to enhance health and fitness. This section will focus on the internal uses of castor oil, suitable dosages, and safety considerations, and recipes for intake.

Internal Uses

Castor oil is well known for its usage as a natural laxative. However, its internal functions extend to boosting detoxification, supporting the immune system, and potentially treating some health issues. The main internal applications for castor oil are as follows:

Natural Laxative

Castor oil is one of the most effective natural laxatives available. It works by stimulating the intestines to transport feces through the bowel, providing relief from constipation.

Mechanism: The principal active ingredient, ricinoleic acid, attaches to receptors on the muscle cells of the intestinal walls, causing them to contract and push feces through the intestines.

Use: To treat constipation, use a tiny quantity of castor oil orally. The normal adult dosage is 1-2 teaspoons, although it is vital to follow prescribed guidelines to avoid any negative effects.

Detoxification

Castor oil can help detoxification processes in the body, especially through its effects on the lymphatic system and liver.

Lymphatic Support: Castor oil helps enhance lymphatic circulation, aiding in the evacuation of toxins and waste from the body. This can increase general immune function and promote detoxification.

Liver Health: Castor oil packs, applied externally over the liver, can help stimulate liver function and facilitate detoxification.

Case Study: Detoxification and Improved Well-being

Mark, a 50-year-old male, suffered low energy levels and regular intestinal problems. His naturopath recommended applying castor oil packs over his liver to help cleansing. Mark administered the packs three times a week for a month. He experienced improved digestion, greater energy levels, and an overall sense of well-being, which he attributed to the enhanced detoxifying process facilitated by castor oil.

Immune System Support

Castor oil has anti-inflammatory and lymphatic drainage properties that help strengthen the immune system. This might be especially helpful when recovering from illness or during the cold and flu season.

In the Case Study, Linda, a 35-year-old teacher, was frequently exposed to colds and other infections at school. She began incorporating castor oil packs into her routine to enhance her immune system. Applying the packs once a week, Linda noted she grew less prone to common diseases and felt more resilient overall.

Dosage and Safety

When taking castor oil internally, it is vital to follow suggested dosages and safety requirements to avoid harmful effects.

Dosage

Laxative Use: For adults, the normal dose is 1-2 tablespoons. For youngsters over the age of 12, a dose of 1-2 tablespoons is generally advised. Always start with a smaller dose to measure your body's response.

Frequency: Castor oil should not be taken as a laxative more than once a week unless prescribed by a healthcare expert. Overuse can develop into dependency and disturb regular bowel function.

Safety Considerations

Pregnancy and Breastfeeding: Pregnant and breastfeeding women should avoid using castor oil internally unless instructed by a healthcare expert. Castor oil can induce uterine contractions, potentially leading to premature labor.

Children: Castor oil should be used with caution in children and only under the advice of a healthcare expert.

Allergies: Although rare, some individuals may have an allergic reaction to castor oil. If you suffer any signs of an allergic response, such as rash, itching, or difficulty breathing, discontinue use and seek medical treatment.

Pre-existing disorders: People with specific health disorders, such as intestinal obstruction, appendicitis, or inflammatory bowel disease, should avoid consuming castor oil internally.

Side Effects

Digestive Discomfort: Some persons may feel cramps, nausea, or diarrhea when taking castor oil as a laxative.

Dehydration: Prolonged use or excessive amounts of castor oil can lead to dehydration and electrolyte abnormalities. Ensure enough hydration when taking castor oil.

Castor Oil Recipes for Consumption

While castor oil is known for its powerful flavor and texture, it can be efficiently blended into numerous recipes to make it more pleasant. Here are 15 unique ways to take castor oil, ensuring you gain its health advantages while enjoying the process.

Castor Oil Shot with Citrus

Ingredients:

- *1 tablespoon castor oil*
- *Juice of half a lemon or orange*

Instructions:

1. Measure 1 tablespoon of castor oil and pour it into a small glass.
2. Squeeze the juice from 1⁄2 a lemon or orange into the glass with the castor oil.
3. Stir vigorously to blend the castor oil and lemon juice.
4. Drink the concoction fast. Follow with a glass of water to help wash it down and further cover the taste.

Benefits:

Digestive Health: Castor oil functions as a natural laxative, aiding in relief from constipation. The citrus juice serves to enhance the flavor and boost digestion with its high vitamin C content.

Immune Support: Lemon or orange juice delivers a dosage of vitamin C, which supports the immune system and helps with overall health.

Detoxification: The combination of castor oil and citrus juice can assist promote detoxification by promoting bowel movements and boosting liver function.

Castor Oil Smoothie

Ingredients:

- *1 tablespoon castor oil*
- *1 cup almond milk (or other milk of choice)*
- *1 banana*
- *1 cup frozen berries*
- *1 tablespoon honey*

Instructions:

1. Add 1 cup of almond milk, 1 banana, and 1 cup of frozen berries into a blender.
2. Blend until smooth.
3. Add 1 tablespoon of castor oil and 1 tablespoon of honey to the blender.
4. To incorporate the castor oil and honey into the smoothie, briefly blend it once more.
5. Enjoy the smoothie right away after pouring it into a glass.

Benefits:

Digestive Health: Castor oil aids in digestion and alleviates constipation, while the banana delivers fiber and helps relax the digestive tract.

Nutrient Boost: The smoothie contains critical vitamins and antioxidants from the berries, and honey adds a natural sweetness with additional health benefits.

Hydration and Energy: Almond milk provides extra nutrients like magnesium and vitamin E while serving as a hydrated base. The smoothie promotes overall wellbeing and increases energy levels.

Ginger and Castor Oil Tea

Ingredients:

- *1 tablespoon castor oil*
- *1 cup hot water*
- *1 tablespoon grated fresh ginger*
- *1 tablespoon honey*

Instructions:

1. Boil 1 cup of water and pour it into a cup or teapot.
2. Add 1 tablespoon of grated fresh ginger to the heated water and let it steep for 5-10 minutes.
3. Strain off the ginger pieces and add 1 tablespoon of castor oil to the ginger tea.
4. Stir in 1 tablespoon of honey for enhanced sweetness and other benefits.
5. Drink the tea while warm.

Benefits:

Digestive Health: The ginger in the tea helps to relax the digestive tract, alleviate nausea, and improve general digestive health. Castor oil produces a moderate laxative effect.

Anti-Inflammatory: Ginger has significant anti-inflammatory characteristics that can help reduce pain and inflammation in the body. The combination with castor oil may boost these effects.

Immune promotion: Honey has antibacterial characteristics and can promote immune function, while ginger strengthens the body's defenses and gives a warming impact.

Castor Oil and Apple Cider Vinegar Tonic

Ingredients:

- *1 tablespoon castor oil*
- *1 tablespoon apple cider vinegar*
- *1 cup warm water*
- *1 teaspoon honey*

Instructions:

1. Warm up one cup of water without bringing it to a boil.
2. Combine one tablespoon of apple cider vinegar and warm water in a glass.
3. Add one teaspoon of honey and one tablespoon of castor oil, and stir.
4. Mix vigorously until the castor oil and honey are entirely combined.
5. Drink the tonic immediately.

Benefits:

Digestive Health: Apple cider vinegar can assist support digestion and balance stomach acids. Combined with castor oil, it can aid in digestion and ease constipation.

Detoxification: Both apple cider vinegar and castor oil are known for their detoxifying effects, helping to drain out toxins from the body.

Metabolism Boost: Apple cider vinegar may assist increase metabolism and promote weight management. The tonic can aid in overall digestive health and energy levels.

Castor Oil and Lemon Detox Drink

Ingredients:

- *1 tablespoon castor oil*
- *Juice of 1 lemon*
- *1 cup warm water*

Instructions:

1. Warm 1 cup of water until it is comfortably warm, but not too hot.
2. Squeeze the juice from 1 lemon into the heating water.
3. Add 1 tablespoon of castor oil to the lemon water.
4. Stir thoroughly to integrate all ingredients.

5. Drink the concoction immediately.

Benefits:

Detoxification: Lemon juice is known for its detoxifying effects and can aid in cleansing the liver. Combined with castor oil, this drink can help stimulate digestion and support detoxification.

Digestive Health: The castor oil provides a gentle laxative effect, while lemon juice aids in digestion and promotes a healthy digestive system.

Immune Support: Lemon juice is rich in vitamin C, which supports the immune system and overall health.

Castor Oil and Honey Elixir

Ingredients:

- *1 tablespoon castor oil*
- *1 tablespoon honey*
- *1 cup warm water*

Instructions:

1. Heat 1 cup of water until warm.
2. In a glass, combine 1 tablespoon of honey with the warm water.
3. Stir in 1 tablespoon of castor oil.
4. Mix well until the castor oil and honey are fully dissolved.

5. Sip the elixir while it's still somewhat warm.

Benefits:

Digestive Health: Honey adds soothing properties and helps to balance the digestive system. Castor oil provides a gentle laxative effect to relieve constipation.

Immune Support: Honey is known for its antimicrobial properties and can help support the immune system, while castor oil offers additional health benefits.

Castor Oil and Mint Tea

Ingredients:

- *1 tablespoon castor oil*
- *1 cup hot water*
- *1 mint tea bag*
- *1 teaspoon honey*

Instructions:

1. Boil 1 cup of water and pour it into a cup.
2. Place the mint tea bag into the hot water and let it steep for 5 minutes.
3. Remove the tea bag and stir in 1 tablespoon of castor oil.
4. Add 1 teaspoon of honey to the tea and mix well.

5. Sip the tea while it's still somewhat warm.

Benefits:

Digestive Health: Mint tea helps soothe the digestive tract and can reduce symptoms of nausea and indigestion. Castor oil provides a mild laxative effect to aid in relieving constipation.

Anti-Inflammatory: Mint has anti-inflammatory properties that can help alleviate inflammation in the digestive system. Combined with castor oil, this tea can support overall digestive health.

Relaxation: Mint tea has a calming effect, which can help reduce stress and promote relaxation, making this tea beneficial for both physical and mental well-being.

Castor Oil and Green Smoothie

Ingredients:

- *1 tablespoon castor oil*
- *1 cup spinach*
- *1 banana*
- *1 cup coconut water*
- *1 tablespoon chia seeds*

Instructions:

1. Add 1 cup of spinach, 1 banana, and 1 cup of coconut water to a blender.
2. Blend until smooth.
3. Add 1 tablespoon of castor oil and 1 tablespoon of chia seeds to the blender.
4. Blend again briefly to combine the ingredients.
5. Enjoy the smoothie right away after pouring it into a glass.

Benefits:

Digestive Health: Spinach and banana both contribute fiber, which supports digestive health. Castor oil adds a gentle laxative effect to help with constipation.

Nutrient Boost: This smoothie is packed with vitamins, minerals, and antioxidants from spinach, banana, and chia seeds. Coconut water adds electrolytes for hydration.

Energy and Vitality: The combination of ingredients helps boost energy levels and provides sustained vitality throughout the day.

Castor Oil and Aloe Vera Juice

Ingredients:

- *1 tablespoon castor oil*
- *1 cup aloe vera juice*
- *Juice of 1 lemon*

Instructions:

1. Pour 1 cup of aloe vera juice into a glass.
2. Squeeze the juice of 1 lemon into the aloe vera juice.
3. Stir in 1 tablespoon of castor oil.
4. Mix well until the castor oil is fully incorporated.
5. Drink the concoction immediately.

Benefits:

Digestive Health: Aloe vera juice is known for its soothing effects on the digestive system and can help with constipation. Castor oil enhances this effect with its mild laxative properties.

Detoxification: Aloe vera and lemon both have detoxifying properties, helping to flush out toxins from the body and support liver health.

Hydration: Aloe vera juice is hydrating and helps maintain proper hydration levels, which is crucial for overall health.

Castor Oil and Carrot Juice

Ingredients:

- *1 tablespoon castor oil*
- *1 cup fresh carrot juice*
- *Juice of 1 orange*

Instructions:

1. Fill a glass with one cup of fresh carrot juice.
2. Squeeze the juice of 1 orange into the carrot juice.
3. Add 1 tablespoon of castor oil.
4. Stir thoroughly to integrate all ingredients.
5. Drink the concoction immediately.

Benefits:

Digestive Health: Carrot juice is rich in vitamins and fiber, which can help support healthy digestion. Castor oil adds a mild laxative effect to aid in relieving constipation.

Nutrient-Rich: Carrot juice provides essential nutrients like vitamin A and beta-carotene, while orange juice adds vitamin C. Together, they support overall health and immune function.

Detoxification: The combination of carrot juice and castor oil can help promote detoxification and support liver function, making this drink beneficial for cleansing the body.

Castor Oil and Turmeric Milk

Ingredients:

- *1 tablespoon castor oil*
- *1 cup warm milk (dairy or plant-based)*
- *1 teaspoon turmeric*

- *1 teaspoon honey*

Instructions:

1. Warm up one cup of milk without boiling it.
2. Add one teaspoon of turmeric and stir until thoroughly mixed.
3. Add 1 tablespoon of castor oil to the milk and stir thoroughly.
4. Sweeten with 1 teaspoon of honey and mix until fully dissolved.
5. When the combination is still warm, drink it.

Benefits:

Anti-Inflammatory: Curcumin, a potent anti-inflammatory found in turmeric, has the ability to lessen pain and inflammation. When used with castor oil, it helps to reduce inflammation all over.

Digestive Health: Both turmeric and castor oil can aid in digestion. Turmeric helps soothe the digestive tract, while castor oil provides a mild laxative effect.

Immune Support: Turmeric and honey both have immune-boosting properties, enhancing the body's defense mechanisms and overall wellness.

Castor Oil and Cucumber Smoothie

Ingredients:

- *1 tablespoon castor oil*
- *1 cucumber*
- *1 apple*
- *1 cup water*
- *Juice of 1 lime*

Instructions:

Combine one apple and one cucumber, peeled and chopped, in a blender.

Pour in one cup of water and one lime's juice into the blender.

Blend until smooth.

Add 1 tablespoon of castor oil and blend briefly to combine.

Enjoy the smoothie right away after pouring it into a glass.

Benefits:

Cucumber and apple both provide dietary fiber, which supports digestive health. Castor oil adds a gentle laxative effect for relief from constipation.

Detoxification: The combination of cucumber, apple, and lime helps to detoxify the body and support overall health.

Castor Oil and Pineapple Juice

Ingredients:

- *1 tablespoon castor oil*
- *1 cup fresh pineapple juice*
- *Juice of 1 lemon*

Instructions:

1. Pour 1 cup of fresh pineapple juice into a glass.
2. Squeeze the juice of 1 lemon into the pineapple juice.
3. Add 1 tablespoon of castor oil and stir well to combine.
4. Drink the concoction immediately.

Benefits:

Bromelain is an enzyme that helps with digestion that can be found in pineapple juice. Castor oil enhances digestive relief with its mild laxative properties.

Immune Support: Pineapple juice is rich in vitamin C, which supports the immune system. The addition of lemon juice further boosts vitamin C intake.

Hydration and Detoxification: Pineapple juice helps with hydration and provides a refreshing, detoxifying effect.

Castor Oil and Beet Juice

Ingredients:

- *1 tablespoon castor oil*
- *1 cup fresh beet juice*
- *Juice of 1 orange*

Instructions:

1. Pour one cup of fresh beet juice into a glass.
2. Squeeze the juice of 1 orange into the beet juice.
3. Add 1 tablespoon of castor oil and stir well to combine.
4. Drink the concoction immediately.

Benefits:

Digestive Health: Beet juice is rich in fiber and minerals that assist digestive health. Castor oil adds a modest laxative effect to assist ease constipation.

Detoxification: Beets are known for their detoxifying effects, boosting liver function and purifying the body. The combination with castor oil aids in detoxifying.

Nutrient-Rich: Beets and oranges give critical vitamins and minerals, including vitamin C and folate, which support general health.

Castor Oil and Herbal Tea Blend

Ingredients:

- *1 tablespoon castor oil*
- *1 cup hot water*
- *1 herbal tea bag (chamomile, peppermint, etc.)*
- *1 teaspoon honey*

Instructions:

1. Boil 1 cup of water and pour it into a cup or teapot.
2. Add 1 herbal tea bag to the hot water and steep for 5 minutes.
3. Take out the tea bag and whisk in 1 teaspoon castor oil.
4. Sip the tea while it is still warm.

Benefits:

Digestive Health: Herbal teas like chamomile and peppermint help ease the digestive system. Castor oil provides further comfort for constipation.

Relaxation: Herbal teas are recognized for their relaxing properties, which can help relieve tension and promote relaxation.

Immune promotion: Honey provides antibacterial characteristics and can promote immune function, making this tea a calming and health-promoting beverage.

Tips for Consumption

Start Small: Begin with a smaller dose, such as 1 teaspoon, to measure your body's response before increasing to 1 tablespoon.

Hydration: Drink plenty of water throughout the day to assist your body absorb the castor oil and avoid dehydration.

Timing: Take castor oil-based drinks in the morning or before bed to fit into your regular schedule and allow time for its benefits.

Mix with Strong Flavors: Combine castor oil with strong flavors like citrus, ginger, or mint to help hide its distinct taste.

External Uses of Castor Oil

Castor oil has a wide range of external uses that can assist the skin, hair, and overall health. Its unique composition allows it to be utilized topically for numerous medicinal and cosmetic objectives. This section will explain the topical applications of castor oil and how to utilize compresses and packs for focused treatment.

Topical Applications

The topical application of castor oil is popular for its hydrating, anti-inflammatory, and therapeutic effects. Here are some common applications:

Skin Care

Moisturizer: Castor oil is a good moisturizer due to its high ricinoleic acid concentration, which helps maintain moisture in the skin. It can be used on its own or blended with other oils like jojoba or almond oil for additional benefits.

Acne Treatment: Castor oil contains antibacterial characteristics that make it useful against acne-causing germs. Its anti-inflammatory qualities can also lessen redness and swelling linked with acne.

Scar and Stretch Mark Reduction: Regular application of castor oil can help minimize the appearance of scars and stretch marks by increasing collagen production and skin regeneration.

Anti-Aging: The antioxidants in castor oil help fight free radicals, which can cause premature aging. Applying castor oil to the face can help minimize the look of fine lines and wrinkles.

Healing Wounds and Burns: Castor oil's antibacterial and anti-inflammatory qualities make it an ideal choice for treating small wounds and burns. It encourages a quicker recovery and aids in infection prevention.

Case Study: Treating Acne with Castor Oil

Jessica, a 25-year-old lady, struggled with severe acne. After reading about the benefits of castor oil, she decided to try it as part of her skincare routine. She put a small bit of castor oil on her face every night before sleeping. Within a few weeks, she saw a considerable reduction in acne and an improvement in her skin's overall texture and appearance.

Hair Care

Hair Growth: Castor oil is thought to encourage hair growth by improving blood circulation to the scalp and giving critical nutrients. Regular application can help decrease hair loss and encourage thicker, healthier hair.

Scalp Health: The antifungal and antibacterial characteristics of castor oil make it beneficial against dandruff and other scalp problems. Using castor oil massages can support the upkeep of a healthy scalp environment.

Moisturizing: Castor oil may deeply moisturize dry and damaged hair, making it smoother, shinier, and more manageable. It can be used as a hot oil therapy or added to conditioners and hair treatments.

Split Ends: Applying castor oil to the ends of the hair can help prevent and mend split ends, minimizing breakage and encouraging healthier hair

Case Study: Promoting Hair Growth with Castor Oil

David, a 30-year-old male with thinning hair, started using castor oil as part of his hair care regimen. Three times a week, he rubbed castor oil into his scalp and left it there all night. After a few months, David observed fresh hair growth and enhanced thickness, making his hair look fuller and healthier.

Nail and Cuticle Care

Cuticle Softener: Castor oil can soften and nourish cuticles, making them easier to handle and less prone to damage. Regular application can help maintain healthy, well-groomed nails.

Strengthening Nails: The minerals in castor oil, particularly vitamin E, can help strengthen brittle and thin nails, minimizing breaking and supporting healthy nail development.

Case Study: Strengthening Nails with Castor Oil

Lily, a 28-year-old lady with brittle nails, started applying castor oil to her nails and cuticles every night before bed. After a few weeks, she noted her nails were stronger, less prone to breaking, and looked better overall.

Compresses and Packs

Compresses and packs are efficient techniques for employing castor oil for focused treatment.

These procedures entail soaking a cloth or pad in castor oil and applying it to a specific area of the body. The warmth and sustained contact allow the oil to enter deeply and deliver therapeutic advantages.

Castor Oil Packs

Castor oil packs are often used for many health conditions, including liver detoxification, pain treatment, and inflammation reduction. How to make and apply a castor oil pack is as follows:

Materials Needed:

Cold-pressed castor oil

A piece of wool or flannel cloth

Plastic wrap

A heating pad or hot water bottle

A towel

Instructions:

1. Soak the Cloth: Pour enough castor oil onto the cloth to saturate it, but not so much that it spills.
2. Apply the Pack: Place the soaking cloth on the desired area (e.g., belly for liver detox, joints for arthritic pain).
3. Cover with Plastic Wrap: Cover the fabric with plastic wrap to keep it in place and avoid stains.

4. Apply Heat: Cover the plastic wrap with a hot water bottle or heating pad. The heat facilitates skin penetration of the castor oil.

5. Relax: Leave the pack on for 30-60 minutes while you relax.

6. wipe Up: After removing the pack, wipe the area with a solution of baking soda and water to eliminate any residual oil.

Benefits of Castor Oil Packs:

Liver Detoxification: Using a castor oil pack on the liver region may assist enhance detoxification and liver function.

Pain Relief: Castor oil packs can relieve pain and inflammation in joints and muscles. They are particularly effective for illnesses like arthritis and muscle strains.

Digestive Health: Castor oil packs can assist improve digestion and treat constipation by stimulating the digestive organs.

Lymphatic System Support: Castor oil packs can promote lymphatic circulation, helping to eliminate toxins and support immunological function.

Case Study: Liver Detoxification with Castor Oil Packs

Anna, a 45-year-old lady, placed castor oil compresses over her liver to promote detoxification. She administered the pack three times a week for a month. Anna reported feeling more energized, experiencing improved digestion, and observed smoother skin, which she ascribed to the cleansing benefits of the castor oil packs.

Castor Oil Compresses

Compresses are comparable to packs but are usually applied to smaller, specific areas. They are excellent for treating injuries, inflammation, and discomfort.

Materials Needed:

Cold-pressed castor oil

A piece of clean cloth or gauze

A plastic bag or wrap

A heating pad or hot water bottle

A towel

Instructions:

1. Soak the Cloth: To soak the cloth, use a sufficient amount of castor oil..

2. Apply the Compress: Place the moistened cloth on the affected area (e.g., a sore muscle, inflamed joint, or wound).

3. Cover with Plastic: Cover the cloth with a plastic bag or wrap to hold it in place.

4. Apply Heat: Place a heating pad or hot water bottle over the compress. The heat helps the castor oil permeate the skin.
5. Relax: Leave the compress on for 20-30 minutes.
6. wipe Up: After removing the compress, wipe the area with a mix of baking soda and water to eliminate any leftover oil.

Benefits of Castor Oil Compresses:

Pain Relief: Compresses can help ease pain from injuries, muscular strains, and joint inflammation.

Wound Healing: Applying a castor oil compress to minor wounds can help avoid infection and aid speedier healing.

Reduction of Inflammation: Compresses can reduce inflammation and swelling in targeted locations, providing relief from ailments including tendinitis and bursitis.

Chapter Five

Castor Oil in Skin Care

Daily Skincare Routine

How to Use:

Cleansing: Use castor oil as part of your oil-cleansing method to remove makeup and impurities. Apply a small amount (a few drops) of castor oil on your face using your fingertips. Massage lightly in circular motions for a few minutes. This helps to dissolve makeup and grime. Rinse with warm water and follow with your usual cleaner if needed.

Moisturizing: Apply a little layer of castor oil to your face and neck after cleaning. You can mix it with other carrier oils, such as almond or jojoba oil, or use it as a stand-alone moisturizer. For a lighter application, blend castor oil with a few drops of your preferred essential oil and gently massage it into your skin.

Toning: For additional advantages, you can add a few drops of castor oil to your toner or face spray. This helps to seal in moisture and deliver a nutritious boost to your skin throughout the day.

Benefits:

Deep Cleansing: Castor oil helps dissolve pollutants and excess sebum from the skin, making it efficient for cleansing.

Rich in fatty acids, castor oil gently hydrates and nourishes the skin, leaving it soft and supple.

Balancing: Regular use of castor oil helps balance skin oils, which can be good for both dry and oily skin types.

2. Treating Acne and Scars

How to Use:

Spot Treatment: For treating acne, apply a small amount of castor oil directly onto the afflicted areas using a clean cotton swab. Apply it overnight, then remove it with a morning wash. Castor oil has antibacterial and anti-inflammatory qualities that help reduce acne and inflammation.

Scar Treatment: To address acne scars, use castor oil on the scarred regions and massage gently for a few minutes. Leave it on overnight or for at least 30 minutes before rinsing off. The oil's high amount of ricinoleic acid stimulates skin regeneration and repair.

Benefits:

Anti-Inflammatory: Castor oil helps reduce inflammation and redness associated with acne.

Antimicrobial: The oil contains natural antibacterial qualities that might help prevent further infection in acne-prone regions.

Scar Healing: Ricinoleic acid in castor oil helps the healing of scars by increasing collagen formation and skin renewal.

3. Moisturizing and Hydrating Tips

How to Use:

Face Mask: Create a moisturizing face mask by mixing 1 tablespoon of castor oil with a few drops of essential oils like lavender or rose. After applying the mixture on your face, let it sit for ten to fifteen minutes. After rinsing with warm water, proceed with your regular skincare regimen.

Overnight Treatment: For deep hydration, apply a liberal layer of castor oil to your face and neck before bedtime. The oil will work overnight to deeply hydrate and heal your skin.

Body Care: Castor oil can also be used to moisturize various sections of the body. Apply it to dry regions such as elbows, knees, and feet. For an additional kick, blend it with your favorite body lotion.

Benefits:

Deep Moisturization: Castor oil hydrates the skin deeply and keeps it hydrated for a long time.

Skin Softening: Regular use helps soften rough spots and smooth the skin's texture.

Barrier Protection: It produces a protective barrier on the skin that helps lock in moisture and keep out environmental contaminants.

4. Anti-Aging Benefits

How to Use:

Serum: Use castor oil as an anti-aging serum by applying a few drops to your face and neck. Gently massage it in using upward strokes. This helps to enhance skin suppleness and decrease the appearance of fine lines and wrinkles.

Eye Care: For the delicate eye area, use a small amount of castor oil to gently massage around the eyes before bed. This helps to moisturize and decrease the look of under-eye wrinkles and puffiness.

Face Cream: Incorporate castor oil into your everyday face cream by pouring a few drops into your regular moisturizer. This increases its moisturizing and anti-aging benefits.

Benefits:

Collagen formation: Castor oil increases collagen and elastin formation, which helps to improve skin firmness and suppleness.

Wrinkle Reduction: Regular usage of castor oil can help minimize the appearance of fine lines and wrinkles by keeping the skin moisturized and encouraging cell renewal.

Skin Regeneration: The oil stimulates the natural repair processes of the skin, helping to decrease indications of aging and preserve a youthful appearance.

Chapter Six

Castor Oil for Hair Care

1. Promoting Hair Growth

How to Use:

Scalp Massage: Warm 1-2 tablespoons of castor oil and apply it directly to your scalp. Use your fingertips to massage the oil into your scalp in circular strokes. This improves blood flow to the hair follicles, stimulating hair growth. If you want a deeper penetration, leave it on for at least 30 minutes or overnight. Rinse with a mild shampoo.

Hair Growth Serum: Mix 1 tablespoon of castor oil with 1 tablespoon of coconut oil or almond oil. Focus on the roots of your hair when applying this mixture to your scalp. You can leave this blend on for 30 minutes before washing it off, which intensifies its nourishing effect.

2. Treating Dry Scalp and Dandruff

How to Use:

Scalp Treatment: Warm 1-2 tablespoons of castor oil and apply it to your scalp. Massage lightly to ensure even distribution. Cover your hair with a shower cap and keep the oil on for at least 30 minutes or overnight for deeper therapy. Wash with a mild shampoo.

Dandruff Relief: Mix 1 tablespoon of castor oil with a few drops of tea tree oil (renowned for its antifungal effects). Apply this mixture to your scalp and keep it on for 30 minutes before rinsing. Tea tree oil helps treat dandruff while castor oil hydrates the scalp.

3. Conditioning and Strengthening Hair

How to Use:

Conditioning Treatment: Apply a sufficient amount of castor oil to damp hair after washing. Focus on the ends to avoid weighing down the roots. Leave it on for 15-30 minutes before rinsing with warm water. For deeper conditioning, put it on overnight.

Strengthening Treatment: Combine one tablespoon each of castor and olive or argan oils. Apply the mixture to your scalp and hair, paying special attention to regions that are brittle. Before washing it off, let it on for thirty to sixty minutes.

Castor Oil and Avocado Mask

Ingredients:

- *1 ripe avocado*
- *1 tablespoon castor oil*
- *1 tablespoon honey*

Instructions:

1. Mash Avocado: Peel and pit the avocado, then mash it in a basin until smooth.
2. Mix Ingredients: Add 1 tablespoon of castor oil and 1 tablespoon of honey to the mashed avocado. Stir until well blended.
3. Apply: Apply the mixture evenly to your hair, focusing on the ends and any dry or damaged areas.
4. Leave On: Give the mask a half-hour to an hour or so.
5. Rinse: Rinse gently with warm water and follow with your regular shampoo.

Uses:

Hydration: Avocado is rich in vitamins and healthy fats that profoundly moisturize and nourish the hair.

Repair: Honey adds moisture and has natural humectant characteristics, which help repair and restore the hair's natural shine.

Softening: This mask helps soften and smoothen hair, making it easier to handle.

Castor Oil and Egg Treatment

Ingredients:

- *1 egg*
- *2 teaspoons castor oil*

Instructions:

1. Prepare Egg Mixture: Beat the egg in a bowl until well blended.
2. Combine Ingredients: Add 2 tablespoons of castor oil to the beaten egg and mix thoroughly.
3. Apply: Starting at the roots and working your way towards the ends, apply the mixture to your hair.
4. Leave On: Allow the treatment to sit for 20-30 minutes.
5. Rinse: Rinse completely with lukewarm water. Steer clear of boiling water as it could cook the egg.

Uses:

Protein Boost: The egg is rich in protein, which strengthens the hair and increases its suppleness.

Nourishment: Castor oil adds moisture and helps trap the nutrients from the egg.

luster: Regular use can boost hair's luster and manageability.

Castor Oil and Coconut Milk Mask

Ingredients:

- *1/4 cup coconut milk*
- *2 teaspoons castor oil*

Instructions:

1. Mix Ingredients: Combine 1/4 cup of coconut milk with 2 tablespoons of castor oil in a bowl.
2. Apply: Apply the mixture evenly to your hair and scalp.
3. Leave On: Leave the mask on for 30 minutes to an hour.
4. Rinse: Rinse well with warm water and shampoo as usual.

Uses:

Moisturizing: Coconut milk delivers deep hydration and nutrients that help moisturize and soften hair.

Strengthening: Castor oil offers nourishing characteristics, encouraging stronger and healthier hair.

Enhancing Shine: This combination promotes shine and smoothness.

Castor Oil and Olive Oil Hair Treatment

Ingredients:

- *2 teaspoons castor oil*
- *2 tablespoons olive oil*

Instructions:

1. Mix Oils: Combine 2 tablespoons of castor oil with 2 teaspoons of olive oil in a bowl.
2. Apply: Apply the mixture to your hair and scalp, focusing on dry or damaged areas.
3. Leave On: Leave the treatment on for 30 minutes.
4. Rinse: Wash out with shampoo and warm water.

Uses

Conditioning: Olive oil provides deep conditioning and adds luster to the hair.

Strengthening: The combination with castor oil helps strengthen hair and minimize breakage.

Hydrating: This treatment helps to replace moisture and maintain hair health.

Castor Oil and Yogurt Hair Mask

Ingredients:

1/2 cup plain yogurt

2 teaspoons castor oil

Instructions:

1. Combine Ingredients: Mix 1/2 cup of plain yogurt with 2 tablespoons of castor oil in a bowl.
2. Apply: Apply the mixture to your hair, ensuring even coverage.
3. Leave On: Let the mask stay for 20-30 minutes.
4. Rinse: Rinse well with warm water and shampoo.

Uses:

Conditioning: Yogurt contains proteins and lactic acid that condition and soften the hair.

Hydration: Castor oil adds moisture, boosting the yogurt's conditioning effects.

Improving Texture: This mask helps improve hair texture and general health.

Castor Oil DIY Hair Masks and Treatments

1. Castor Oil and Aloe Vera Mask

Ingredients:

- *2 teaspoons castor oil*
- *2 teaspoons aloe vera gel*

Instructions:

1. Mix Ingredients: In a bowl, blend 2 tablespoons of castor oil with 2 tablespoons of fresh aloe vera gel. Once the mixture is uniformly smooth, give it a good stir
2. Apply: Apply the mixture to your hair and scalp, ensuring even coverage. Focus on regions that are extremely dry or damaged.
3. Leave On: Allow the mask to rest for 30 minutes to let the ingredients penetrate deeply.
4. Rinse: Use warm water to completely rinse, then use your usual shampoo.

Uses:

Hydration: Aloe vera gives deep hydration and calms the scalp, while castor oil locks in moisture.

Healing: Aloe vera offers healing characteristics that can aid with scalp ailments such as dryness or inflammation.

Shine: This mask promotes hair shine and smoothness, leaving hair looking healthy and bright.

2. Castor Oil and Banana Hair Mask

Ingredients:

- *1 ripe banana*
- *2 teaspoons castor oil*

Instructions

1. Prepare Banana: Peel and mash the ripe banana in a bowl until smooth.
2. Combine Ingredients: Mix the mashed banana with 2 teaspoons of castor oil until fully blended.
3. Apply: Apply the mixture to your hair, focusing on the ends and any dry areas.
4. Leave On: Let the mask stay for 20-30 minutes.
5. Rinse: Rinse gently with warm water and wash as needed.

Uses:

Nourishment: Bananas are rich in vitamins and minerals that nourish and build the hair.

Moisture: Castor oil gives more moisture, making the hair smoother and more manageable

3. Castor Oil and Honey Hair Mas

Ingredients:

- *2 teaspoons castor oil*
- *2 tablespoons honey*

Instructions:

1. Mix Ingredients: Combine 2 teaspoons of castor oil with 2 tablespoons of honey in a bowl. Stir until the mixture is smooth.
2. Apply: Apply the mixture evenly to your hair, focusing on the ends and dry patches.
3. Leave On: Put the mask on and wait thirty minutes.
4. Rinse: Rinse with warm water and wash to eliminate any residue.

Uses:

Deep Moisturization: Honey is a natural humectant that attracts moisture, and castor oil amplifies this hydrating action.

Shine: The mixture gives shine and softness to the hair.

Repair: Honey helps repair and renew damaged hair, while castor oil strengthens it.

4. Castor Oil and Green Tea Treatment

Ingredients:

- *1/2 cup brewed green tea (cooled)*
- *2 teaspoons castor oil*

Instructions:

1. Prepare Green Tea: Brew a cup of green tea and let it cool to room temperature.
2. Mix Ingredients: Combine 1/2 cup of cooled green tea with 2 tablespoons of castor oil in a bowl.
3. Apply: Apply the mixture to your hair and scalp.
4. Leave On: Let it sit for 30 minutes.
5. Rinse: Rinse well with warm water and shampoo.

Uses:

Antioxidant Benefits: Green tea is rich in antioxidants that assist in preserving the hair and scalp from damage.

Strengthening: Castor oil adds nutrients and helps strengthen hair.

Scalp Health: This therapy fosters a healthy scalp environment, potentially minimizing concerns like dandruff.

5. Castor Oil and Shea Butter Mask

Ingredients:

- *2 teaspoons castor oil*
- *2 tablespoons shea butter*

Instructions:

1. Melt Shea Butter: Gently melt the shea butter using a double boiler or microwave. Allow it to cool somewhat.
2. Combine Ingredients: Mix the melted shea butter with 2 teaspoons of castor oil until smooth.
3. Apply: Apply the mixture to your hair and scalp, focusing on dry or damaged areas.
4. Leave On: Leave the mask on for 30 minutes.
5. Wash Out: Wash out completely with shampoo and warm water.

Uses:

Deep Conditioning: Shea butter delivers deep conditioning, while castor oil increases the nourishing properties.

restore and Strengthen: This mask helps to restore damaged hair and strengthen it from the roots.

Moisture seal: Both chemicals seal in moisture, increasing hair texture and avoiding dryness.

Chapter Seven

Castor Oil for Nails and Cuticles

1. Strengthening Nails

How to Use:

Direct Application: Apply a small amount of castor oil straight onto your nails and nail beds. Gently massage the oil into the nail surface and surrounding skin for a few minutes. This technique promotes blood circulation and nourishes the nails.

Soak Method: Fill a small bowl with a mixture of castor oil and a few drops of lemon juice. Soak your nails in this solution for around 10-15 minutes. Lemon juice helps to lighten the nails while castor oil strengthens them.

Nail Strengthening Treatment: Combine 1 tablespoon of castor oil with 1 teaspoon of vitamin E oil. Apply this mixture to your nails and cuticles before bed, and let it on overnight. This treatment gives intense hydration and nutrients.

2. Moisturizing Cuticles

How to Use:

Cuticle Oil: Use a little brush or your fingers to apply castor oil directly to your cuticles. Gently massage the oil into the cuticles and the surrounding skin. Do this every day to maintain soft and hydrated cuticles.

Cuticle Soak: Mix equal parts castor oil and almond oil. Soak your fingers in this combination for 10 minutes to soften and hydrate the cuticles. After soaking, carefully push back the cuticles with a cuticle pusher.

DIY Cuticle Cream: Create a cuticle cream by mixing 1 tablespoon of castor oil with 1 tablespoon of shea butter. Your cuticles and nails should be rubbed with the lotion after application. During dry seasons, this rich cream is extremely nice.

3. Home Manicure Tips

How to Use:

Nail Prep: Before commencing your manicure, apply castor oil to your nails and cuticles to soften them. Gently press back the cuticles with a cuticle pusher and clip any extra cuticle. This ensures a clean and smooth nail surface.

Nail Strengthening Treatment: After filing and shaping your nails, apply a thin layer of castor oil to the entire nail surface and cuticles. Massage in circular strokes to allow the oil to permeate. This procedure is useful for strengthening nails and preparing them for polish.

Cuticle Care: During your home manicure, periodically use castor oil to maintain cuticle health. Apply it after removing the nail paint and before applying a new coat. This helps keep cuticles hydrated and prevents them from drying out.

Special Applications of Castor Oil

1. Healing Minor Wounds and Infections

How to Use:

Clean the region: Before applying castor oil, clean the affected region with gentle soap and water to eliminate any dirt or debris. Pat dry with a clean towel.

Put Castor Oil: Using a sterile cotton ball or swab put a tiny amount of castor oil directly onto the minor wound or infection. Make sure the oil covers the entire afflicted region.

Cover: Cover the area with sterile gauze or bandages to provide additional protection and to help hold the oil in place. This lets the oil work while protecting the wound from dirt and bacteria.

Reapply: Reapply the castor oil and replace the bandage 1-2 times a day, depending on the severity of the wound. Continue until the wound has healed.

2. Relieving Joint Pain and Muscle Aches

How to Use:

Prepare the Oil: Warm a tiny amount of castor oil by placing the bottle in warm water or microwaving it for a few seconds. Do not overheat; the oil should be comfortably warm to the touch.

Massage: Apply the warm castor oil straight to the injured joint or muscle. Massage the oil into the skin with light, circular strokes. This improves the absorption of the oil and increases blood flow.

Place a Heat Source: For deeper relief, you can place a heating pad or warm towel over the region after applying the oil. The heat helps to permeate the oil farther into the tissues.

Repeat: Apply the castor oil therapy 1-2 times daily or as needed to ease pain and discomfort.

3. Enhancing Eyelash and Eyebrow Growth

How to Use:

Clean the Area: Ensure that your face is clean and free from makeup. Wash your face gently, then pat it dry.

Apply Castor Oil: Use a clean mascara brush or a cotton swab to apply a tiny amount of castor oil to your eyelashes and eyebrows. Be careful to avoid getting the oil in your eyes.

Uniform Application: For eyelashes, brush the oil along the base of the lashes and achieve uniform distribution. For eyebrows, apply the oil directly to the brow area and lightly massage it in.

Leave On: Allow the oil to remain on your eyelashes and eyebrows overnight for the best benefits. Rinse off with warm water in the morning if preferred.

Regular Use: Apply the oil nightly for consistent effects. It may take many weeks to detect benefits in hair growth.

4. Soothing Sunburn

How to Use:

Clean the Area: Gently wash the burnt skin with cool water and mild soap to eliminate any contaminants. Pat dry with a gentle towel.

Apply Castor Oil: Pour a tiny amount of castor oil into your palm and gently apply it to the tanned region. You can also use a cotton ball or pad for application.

Massage Gently: Massage the oil into the skin using gentle, circular strokes. This helps the oil absorb better and lessens irritation.

Reapply: Apply the castor oil 2-3 times a day as needed to calm the skin and eliminate irritation.

5. Treating Dry and Cracked Heels

How to Use:

Prepare the Feet: Wash your feet properly and dry them fully. If desired, bathe your feet in warm, soapy water for 10 minutes to soften the skin.

Apply Castor Oil: Apply a sufficient amount of castor oil to the dry and cracked parts of your heels. Apply with a cotton ball or your fingertips.

Cover: For optimal results, cover your feet with cotton socks to assist the oil stay in place and prevent it from rubbing off.

Leave On: Leave the castor oil on overnight to allow it to deeply enter and hydrate the skin.

Repeat: Apply castor oil nightly to retain softness and prevent further cracking.

6. Reducing Stretch Marks

How to Use:

Clean the region: Ensure the region with stretch marks is clean and dry.

Apply Castor Oil: Gently massage castor oil into the stretch marks using circular motions. Apply enough oil to cover the marks fully.

Leave On: Allow the oil to linger on the skin. You can also use a plastic wrap or bandage to keep the oil in place for a more intense treatment.

Repeat: Apply the oil daily, ideally before bedtime, for the best benefits. It may take many weeks to detect improvements.

7. Easing Menstrual Cramps

How to Use:

Warm the Oil: Slightly warm castor oil by placing the bottle in warm water or microwaving it for a few seconds.

Apply: Gently massage the heated castor oil onto your lower abdomen where you suffer menstruation pains.

Use a Heating Pad: For increased relief, place a heating pad or warm towel over the region after applying the oil. The combined warmth promotes improved circulation and helps to relax the muscles.

Repeat: Apply the oil and use the heating pad 2-3 times a day as needed for relief during menstrual periods.

8. Treating Eczema and Psoriasis

How to Use:

Clean the Area: Gently clean the afflicted skin areas with mild soap and water. Pat dry with a gentle towel.

Apply Castor Oil: Apply a thin layer of castor oil straight to the eczema or psoriasis spots. Use a cotton ball or your fingertips for application.

Massage Gently: Rub the oil into the skin with gentle, circular strokes to ensure uniform covering.

Cover: For more severe therapy, cover the area with a bandage or gauze to keep the oil from rubbing off and to allow it to stay in place.

Repeat: Apply castor oil 2-3 times a day, or as needed, to help manage symptoms.

9. Alleviating Headaches

How to Use:

Warm the Oil: Slightly warm castor oil by placing the bottle in warm water or microwaving it for a few seconds. Ensure it is comfortably warm to avoid burns.

Apply to Temples: Using your fingertips, apply a tiny amount of heated castor oil to your temples and the base of your neck. Gently massage in circular strokes.

Rest: After application, rest in a calm, comfortable position for 15-20 minutes to enable the oil to operate.

Repeat: Use this approach as needed to relieve headache symptoms.

10. Reducing Varicose Veins

How to Use:

Prepare the Oil: Warm a small amount of castor oil gently. This helps improve its absorption.

Apply to Affected Areas: Gently massage the warmed oil onto the varicose veins and surrounding areas using upward strokes. This approach stimulates greater blood flow.

Use Compression: For extra benefit, cover the treated region with a compression bandage or wear compression stockings after applying the oil.

Repeat: Apply castor oil regularly, ideally at night, to help manage symptoms.

11. Soothing and Hydrating Chapped Lips

How to Use:

Clean Lips: Gently clean your lips with water to eliminate any debris or residue.

Apply Castor Oil: Use a clean fingertip or a small brush to apply a thin layer of castor oil directly to your lips.

Reapply: Apply the oil as needed throughout the day, especially after eating or drinking, to retain hydration.

Overnight Treatment: For intensive hydration, apply a liberal layer of castor oil to your lips before bed and keep it on overnight.

Chapter Eight

Castor Oil Recipes and DIY Projects

Homemade Castor Oil Soaps

These recipes are beginner-friendly and convenient, as they utilize pre-made soap bases that you melt and personalize.

1. Castor Oil and Lavender Melt-and-Pour Soap

Ingredients:

- *1 pound clear or white melt-and-pour soap base*
- *1 tablespoon castor oil*
- *10-15 drops of lavender essential oil*
- *Dried lavender buds (optional)*

Instructions:

1. Melt the Soap Base: Cut the soap base into small pieces and melt it in a microwave-safe bowl or double boiler.
2. Add Castor Oil: Once melted, whisk in the castor oil.
3. Add Essential Oil: Mix in the lavender essential oil.
4. Pour into Molds: Fill molds with the mixture.
5. Add Dried Lavender: Sprinkle dried lavender buds on top if desired.
6. Let it Set: Allow the soap to cool and solidify for several hours before removing it from the molds.

Benefits:

Lavender Essential Oil: Known for its calming and relaxing characteristics.

Castor Oil: Adds more hydration and conditioning.

2. Castor Oil and Coconut Milk Soap

Ingredients:

- *1 lb white melt-and-pour soap base*
- *1 tablespoon castor oil*
- *1/4 cup coconut milk*
- *5-10 drops vanilla essential oil (optional)*

Instructions:

1. Melt the Soap Base: The soap base should be melted in a double boiler or microwave-safe basin.
2. Incorporate Castor Oil and Coconut Milk: Stir in the castor oil and coconut milk.
3. Add Fragrance: Mix with the vanilla essential oil if using.
4. Pour into Molds: Fill molds with the mixture.
5. Cool and Harden: Give the soap several hours to cool and solidify.

Benefits:

Coconut Milk: Provides extra moisturizing and calming effects.

Castor Oil: Enhances the soap's lather and conditioning.

3. Castor Oil and Oatmeal Soap

Ingredients:

*   *1-pound clear melt-and-pour soap base*
*   *1 tablespoon castor oil*
*   *1/4 cup finely ground oatmeal*
*   *5-10 drops honey fragrance oil (optional)*

Instructions:

1. Melt the Soap Base: The soap base should be melted in a double boiler or microwave-safe basin.
2. Add Castor Oil and Oatmeal: Stir in the castor oil and finely ground oatmeal.
3. Add Fragrance: Mix with honey fragrance oil if desired.
4. Pour into Molds: Pour into soap molds.
5. Let it Set: Allow it to cool and harden entirely.

Benefits:

Oatmeal: Provides gentle exfoliating and soothing effects.

Castor Oil: Adds a moisturizing effect.

4. Castor Oil with Green Tea Soap

Ingredients:

*   *1 lb white melt-and-pour soap base*
*   *1 tablespoon castor oil*
*   *2 tablespoons brewed green tea (cooled)*
*   *5-10 drops green tea fragrance oil (optional)*

Instructions:

1. Melt the Soap Base: The soap base should be melted in a double boiler or microwave-safe basin.

2. Add Castor Oil and Green Tea: Stir in the castor oil and brewed green tea.

3. Add Fragrance: Mix in green tea fragrance oil if using.

4. Pour into Molds: Pour into soap molds.

5. Cool and Harden: Let the soap set for many hours.

Benefits:

Green Tea: Provides antioxidant qualities and soothes the skin.

Castor Oil: Enhances hydration.

5. Castor Oil and Honey Soap

Ingredients:

- *1-pound clear melt-and-pour soap base*
- *1 tablespoon castor oil*
- *2 tablespoons honey*
- *5-10 drops almond fragrance oil (optional)*

Instructions:

1. Melt the Soap Base: The soap base should be melted in a double boiler or microwave-safe basin.

2. Mix in Castor Oil and Honey: Stir in the castor oil and honey.

3. Add Fragrance: Add almond fragrance oil as desired.

4. Pour into Molds: Fill molds with the mixture.

5. Let it Set: Let it cool and get solid.

Benefits:

Honey: Provides moisturizing and antimicrobial effects.

Castor Oil: Adds conditioning and moisture.

6. Castor Oil and Aloe Vera Soap

Ingredients:

1 lb white melt-and-pour soap base

1 tablespoon castor oil

2 teaspoons aloe vera gel

5-10 drops cucumber fragrance oil (optional)

Instructions:

1. Melt the Soap Base: The soap base should be melted in a double boiler or microwave-safe basin.

2. Incorporate Castor Oil and Aloe Vera: Add the aloe vera gel and castor oil, and stir.

3. Add Fragrance: Mix in cucumber fragrance oil if using.

4. Pour into Molds: Pour into molds.

5. Cool and Harden: Let the soap cool and harden.

Benefits:

Aloe Vera: Soothes and moisturizes the skin.

Castor Oil: Adds hydration and conditioning.

7. Castor Oil and Shea Butter Soap

Ingredients:

- *1-pound clear melt-and-pour soap base*
- *1 tablespoon castor oil*
- *1/4 cup shea butter*
- *5-10 drops vanilla or almond fragrance oil (optional)*

Instructions:

1. Melt the Soap Base: The soap base should be melted in a double boiler or microwave-safe basin.
2. Add Castor Oil and Shea Butter: Stir in the castor oil and shea butter.
3. Add Fragrance: Add vanilla or almond fragrance oil if desired.
4. Pour into Molds: Pour into soap molds.
5. Cool and Harden: Let the soap set for many hours.

Benefits:

Shea Butter: Provides great moisturization and skin nourishment.

Castor Oil: Enhances lather and conditioning.

8. Castor Oil with Peppermint Soap

Ingredients:

- *1 lb white melt-and-pour soap base*
- *1 tablespoon castor oil*
- *10-15 drops of peppermint essential oil*
- *Dried peppermint leaves (optional)*

Instructions:

1. Melt the Soap Base: The soap base should be melted in a double boiler or microwave-safe basin.
2. Add Castor Oil and Peppermint: Stir in the castor oil and peppermint essential oil.
3. Add Peppermint Leaves: Sprinkle dried peppermint leaves into the molds if desired.
4. Pour into Molds: Fill molds with the mixture.
5. Cool and Harden: Allow the soap to solidify and cool.

Benefits:

Peppermint Essential Oil: Provides a refreshing and revitalizing impact.

Castor Oil: Adds moisture and increases lather.

9. Castor Oil and Carrot Soap

Ingredients:

- *1-pound clear melt-and-pour soap base*
- *1 tablespoon castor oil*
- *1/4 cup carrot puree (cooled)*
- *5-10 drops of carrot seed essential oil (optional)*

Instructions:

1. Melt the Soap Base: The soap base should be melted in a double boiler or microwave-safe basin.
2. Add Castor Oil and Carrot Puree: Stir in the castor oil and carrot puree.
3. Add Essential Oil: Mix with carrot seed essential oil if using.
4. Pour into Molds: Fill molds with the mixture.
5. Cool and Harden: To help the soap harden, let it cool.

Benefits:

Carrot Puree: Rich in vitamins and antioxidants.

Castor Oil: Enhances hydration and conditioning.

10. Castor Oil and Rose Clay Soap

Ingredients:

- *1 lb white melt-and-pour soap base*
- *1 tablespoon castor oil*
- *2 tablespoons rose clay*
- *5-10 drops rose scent oil (optional)*

Instructions:

1. Melt the Soap Base: The soap base should be melted in a double boiler or microwave-safe basin.
2. Mix in Castor Oil and Rose Clay: Stir in the castor oil and rose clay.
3. Add Fragrance: Add rose fragrance oil as desired.
4. Pour into Molds: Fill molds with the mixture.
5. Cool and Harden: Let the soap set and harden.

Benefits:

Rose Clay: Provides moderate exfoliation and improves skin texture.

Castor Oil: Adds more hydration and conditioning.

Relaxing Lavender Blend

Ingredients:

- *2 teaspoons castor oil*
- *10 drops of lavender essential oil*
- *5 drops of chamomile essential oil*

Instructions:

1. Mix the castor oil and essential oils in a clean glass bottle.
2. Shake well to mix.
3. Apply a tiny quantity to your wrists, neck, or temples, and gently massage in.

Benefits:

1. Lavender Essential Oil: It helps reduce tension and anxiety and is well-known for these soothing and relaxing qualities. and anxiety.
2. Chamomile Essential Oil: Adds relaxing qualities, which can help with sleep and relaxation.
3. Castor Oil: Provides a hydrating basis and helps in the absorption of essential oils.

2. Energizing Citrus Blend

Ingredients:

- *2 teaspoons castor oil*
- *5 drops of orange essential oil*
- *5 drops of lemon essential oil*
- *5 drops of grapefruit essential oil*

Instructions:

1. Combine the castor oil with the essential oils in a glass bottle.
2. Shake thoroughly to combine.
3. Apply to the pulse points or put in a diffuser for an invigorating boost.

Benefits:

Orange, Lemon, and Grapefruit Essential Oils: These citrus oils are known for their uplifting and invigorating qualities, boosting positivity and mental clarity.

Castor Oil: Acts as a carrier oil, allowing the essential oils to be applied to the skin or diffused efficiently.

3. Calming Mint Blend

Ingredients:

- *2 teaspoons castor oi*
- *6 drops peppermint essential oil*
- *4 drops of spearmint essential oil*
- *4 drops of lavender essential oil*

Instructions:

1. Blend the castor oil and essential oils in a glass jar.

2. Shake well before each use.

3. Apply on the back of the neck, and temples, or use in a diffuser to refresh and calm.

Benefits:

Peppermint & Spearmint Essential Oils: Provide a cooling sensation and aid in alleviating mental tiredness and increase concentration.

Lavender Essential Oil: Adds relaxing qualities to complement the energizing mint oils.

Castor Oil: Helps soothe and calm the skin while improving the blend's effectiveness.

4. Soothing Sleep Blend

Ingredients:

- *2 teaspoons castor oil*
- *8 drops of cedarwood essential oil*
- *6 drops sandalwood essential oil*
- *4 drops of bergamot essential oil*

Instructions:

1. Mix the castor oil and essential oils in a glass bottle.
2. Shake to blend.
3. Apply on the bottoms of your feet or use a diffuser before bedtime.

Benefits:

Cedarwood and Sandalwood Essential Oils: Promote relaxation and provide a quiet environment suitable for sleep.

Bergamot Essential Oil: Helps reduce tension and anxiety, facilitating peaceful sleep.

Castor Oil: Provides a nutritious basis that assists the essential oils to be absorbed properly.

5. Detoxifying Blend

Ingredients:

- *2 teaspoons castor oil*
- *7 drops of lemon essential oil*
- *7 drops juniper berry essential oil*
- *6 drops rosemary essential oil*

Instructions:

1. Combine castor oil with the essential oils in a clean glass bottle.
2. Shake thoroughly to combine.
3. Apply to regions of the body that feel tense or use a diffuser to help with cleansing.

Benefits:

Lemon Essential Oil: Supports cleansing and enhances mood.

Juniper Berry Essential Oil: Known for its cleansing effects and helps to reduce tension.

Rosemary Essential Oil: Enhances mental clarity and helps with physical weariness.

Castor Oil: Enhances the detoxifying benefits and provides a calming basis.

6. Mood-Lifting Floral Blend

Ingredients:

- *2 teaspoons castor oil*
- *5 drops of rose essential oil*
- *5 drops of geranium essential oil*
- *5 drops ylang-ylang essential oil*

Instructions:

1. Mix the castor oil with the essential oils in a glass container.
2. Shake to blend.
3. Apply on the chest and shoulders or use a diffuser to enhance mood.

Benefits:

Rose Essential Oil: Promotes emotional balance and increases mood.

Geranium Essential Oil: Helps with stress alleviation and emotional stability.

Ylang-Ylang Essential Oil: Adds a sweet, floral scent that aids in relaxation and emotional upliftment.

Castor Oil: Acts as a carrier oil to facilitate proper application and absorption.

7. Invigorating Spice Blend

Ingredients:

- *2 teaspoons castor oil*
- *6 drops cinnamon essential oil*
- *5 drops of clove essential oil*
- *4 drops of ginger essential oil*

Instructions:

1. Combine the castor oil with the essential oils in a glass bottle.
2. Shake thoroughly to combine.
3. Apply on the lower back or put in a diffuser to excite and rejuvenate.

Benefits:

Cinnamon and Clove Essential Oils: Provide a warming sensation and excite the senses.

Ginger Essential Oil: Adds a spicy note that energizes and helps mental clarity.

Castor Oil: Provides a relaxing foundation and improves the absorption of essential oils.

8. Stress-Relief Blend

Ingredients:

- 2 teaspoons castor oil
- 8 drops of frankincense essential oil
- 6 drops of myrrh essential oil
- 4 drops of lavender essential oil

Instructions:

1. Blend castor oil and essential oils in a clean glass bottle.
2. Shake to blend.
3. Apply to pulse points, and neck, or use a diffuser to ease stress.

Benefits:

Frankincense & Myrrh Essential Oils: Known for their grounding and relaxing characteristics, these oils help relieve stress and promote relaxation.

Lavender Essential Oil: Enhances the relaxing benefits of the combination.

Castor Oil: Enhances the therapeutic effects and provides a moisturizing basis.

9. Focus and Clarity Blend

Ingredients:

- *2 teaspoons castor oil*
- *6 drops of basil essential oil*
- *5 drops peppermint essential oil*
- *5 drops of rosemary essential oil*

Instructions:

Mix castor oil with the essential oils in a glass jar.

Shake thoroughly to combine.

Apply to the temples, and neck, or use in a diffuser to increase focus and mental clarity.

Benefits:

Basil and Rosemary Essential Oils: Improve focus and mental clarity.

Peppermint Essential Oil: Provides a refreshing effect that helps to relieve brain fog.

Castor Oil: Acts as a carrier oil and facilitates the absorption of essential oils.

10. Revitalizing Blen

Ingredients:

- *2 teaspoons castor oil*
- *7 drops eucalyptus essential oil*
- *7 drops of tea tree essential oil*
- *6 drops peppermint essential oil*

Instructions:

1. Combine castor oil with the essential oils in a glass bottle.

2. Shake thoroughly to combine.

3. Apply to the chest, or back, or use a diffuser to invigorate and refresh.

Benefits:

Eucalyptus and Tea Tree Essential Oils: Provide a cleansing and invigorating effect, helping to cleanse respiratory passageways.

Peppermint Essential Oil: Adds an energizing touch that stimulates the senses.

Castor Oil: Enhances the rejuvenating benefits and provides a calming basis.

Refreshing Citrus Mint Blend

Ingredients:

- *2 teaspoons castor oil*
- *5 drops peppermint essential oil*
- *5 drops of lime essential oil*
- *5 drops of basil essential oil*

Instructions:

1. Mix the castor oil and essential oils in a glass bottle.

2. Shake well to mix.

3. Use in a diffuser or apply to pulse points for a revitalizing and rejuvenating effect.

Benefits:

Peppermint Essential Oil: Rejuvenating and refreshing effect that awakens the senses.

Lime Essential Oil: Uplifts and revitalizes, imparting a zesty tone.

Basil Essential Oil: Enhances mental clarity and attention.

Castor Oil: Acts as a carrier oil, assisting in the absorption of essential oils.

2. Grounding Woodsy Blend

Ingredients:

- *2 teaspoons castor oil*
- *6 drops of cedarwood essential oil*
- *6 drops sandalwood essential oil*
- *4 drops of vetiver essential oil*

Instructions:

1. Combine the castor oil with the essential oils in a clean glass bottle.

2. Shake thoroughly to combine.

3. Apply to the wrists, and neck, or put in a diffuser to produce a grounding and peaceful ambiance.

4. Benefits:

5. Cedarwood and Sandalwood Essential Oils: Provide grounding and relaxing qualities, creating a sense of stability.

6. Vetiver Essential Oil: Known for its rich, earthy aroma that assists with relaxation and stress relief.

7. Castor Oil: Enhances the calming benefits and provides a hydrating basis.

3. Invigorating Spice Blend

Ingredients

- *2 teaspoons castor oil*
- *5 drops cinnamon essential oil*
- *5 drops of clove essential oil*
- *5 drops of ginger essential oil*

Instructions:

1. Mix the castor oil with the essential oils in a glass bottle.
2. Shake well to mix.
3. Apply on the lower back, or chest, or use in a diffuser for an energizing and warming effect
4. Benefits:
5. Cinnamon and Clove Essential Oils: Provide warming and invigorating effects that increase energy levels.
6. Ginger Essential Oil: Adds a spicy, energizing touch that aids with mental clarity.
7. Castor Oil: Acts as a carrier oil, distributing the essential oils efficiently.

4. Harmonizing Floral Blend

Ingredients:

- *2 teaspoons castor oil*
- *5 drops of rose essential oil*
- *5 drops of geranium essential oil*
- *5 drops ylang-ylang essential oil*

Instructions:

1. Combine the castor oil with the essential oils in a glass bottle.
2. Shake thoroughly to combine.
3. Apply to the pulse points or use a diffuser to produce a harmonious and uplifting atmosphere.

Benefits:

Rose Essential Oil: Known for its emotionally balanced effects and fostering self-love.

Geranium Essential Oil: Enhances emotional equilibrium and lowers stress.

Ylang-Ylang Essential Oil: Adds a lovely flowery fragrance that assists with relaxation and mood-boosting.

Castor Oil: Provides a nutritious basis that assists the essential oils to be absorbed properly.

5. Clearing Breathe Blend

Ingredients:

- *2 teaspoons castor oil*
- *6 drops of eucalyptus essential oil*
- *5 drops of tea tree essential oil*
- *4 drops of rosemary essential oil*

Instructions:

1. Mix the castor oil with the essential oils in a clean glass bottle.
2. Shake well to mix.
3. Apply to the chest and throat area, or use a diffuser to improve respiratory health.

Benefits:

Eucalyptus & Tea Tree Essential Oils: Provide cleansing and invigorating benefits, helping to open nasal passages and aid breathing.

Rosemary Essential Oil: Adds a stimulating touch that helps respiratory function and mental clarity.

Castor Oil: Helps to soothe and hydrate, boosting the therapeutic effects of the essential oils.

Infused Castor Oil for Enhanced Benefits

Infused castor oil is a potent version of conventional castor oil that combines the benefits of castor oil with the therapeutic characteristics of numerous herbs, flowers, and other botanicals. This technique involves steeping or infusing plant materials in castor oil to extract their active ingredients, resulting in a more versatile and potent product. Here's an in-depth look into infused castor oil, including procedures, advantages, and popular infusions.

What is Infused Castor Oil?

Infused castor oil is manufactured by mixing castor oil with various herbs or botanical compounds to increase its therapeutic qualities. The infusion process absorbs beneficial chemicals from the plant materials, enhancing the castor oil with more nutrients, essential oils, and active substances. This improved oil can then be used for a number of health and beauty applications.

Methods for Infusing Castor Oil

1. Cold Infusion

Method:

Select Ingredients: Choose dried herbs, flowers, or botanicals such as chamomile, lavender, or rosemary. Ensure the ingredients are thoroughly dry to prevent mold formation.

Prepare the Jar: Sterilize a glass jar with a tight-fitting cover.

Combine Ingredients: Fill the jar with your chosen dry herbs and cover them with castor oil.

Infuse: Seal the jar tightly and set it in a cold, dark spot for 2-4 weeks. Shake the container every day to help the infusion process.

Filter: After the infusion period, filter the oil using a fine mesh strainer or cheesecloth to remove the plant residue. Pour the infused oil into a dark, spotless glass bottle.

Benefits:

Gentle Extraction: Cold infusion retains the delicate characteristics of the herbs and maintains the purity of the castor oil.

Simple Process: Requires minimal equipment and may be done at home with ease.

2. Warm Infusion

Method:

Select Ingredients: Choose dry herbs or botanicals.

Prepare the Jar: Sterilize a glass jar and place the dried materials inside.

Combine Ingredients: Cover the herbs with castor oil.

Warm Infusion: Place the jar in a double boiler or slow cooker on low heat for 1-3 hours. Maintain a low temperature to avoid overheating the oil.

Cool and Strain: Let the oil cool before filtering out the plant material. Pour the infused oil into a dark, spotless glass bottle.

Benefits:

Faster Infusion: The warmth speeds up the extraction of active components from the plants.

Enhanced Aroma: Provides a more intense infusion, which might result in a stronger aroma and more prominent effects.

Popular Infusions and Their Benefits

1. Lavender Infused Castor Oil

Ingredients:

- *2 teaspoons dried lavender flowers*
- *1 cup castor oil*

Instructions:

1. Combine dried lavender and castor oil in a sterilized glass container.
2. Infuse using the cold or warm approach for 2-4 weeks.
3. Strain and store in a dark bottle.

Benefits:

Lavender Essential Oil: Known for its calming and relaxing characteristics. Lavender-infused castor oil is fantastic for encouraging relaxation, facilitating sleep, and relaxing the skin.

2. Chamomile Infused Castor Oil

Ingredients:

- *2 teaspoons dried chamomile flowers*
- *1 cup castor oil*

Instructions:

1. Combine dried chamomile and castor oil in a sterilized glass jar.
2. Infuse for 2-4 weeks using the cold or heated technique.
3. Strain and store in a dark bottle.

Benefits:

Chamomile Essential Oil: Provides anti-inflammatory and relaxing characteristics, making it great for calming inflamed skin and supporting general skin health.

3. Rosemary Infused Castor Oil

Ingredients:

- *2 teaspoons dried rosemary leaves*
- *1 cup castor oil*

Instructions:

1. In a sterile jar, mix castor oil and dried rosemary.
2. Infuse for 2-4 weeks using the cold or heated technique.
3. Strain and transfer to a dark bottle.

Benefits:

Rosemary Essential Oil: Known for its energizing and revitalizing effects. Rosemary-infused castor oil can boost hair growth, improve scalp health, and excite the senses.

4. Calendula Infused Castor Oil

Ingredients:

- *2 teaspoons dried calendula petals*
- *1 cup castor oil*

Instructions:

1. Combine dried calendula and castor oil in a sterilized jar.
2. Infuse for 2-4 weeks using the cold or heated technique.
3. Strain and store in a dark bottle.

Benefits:

Calendula Essential Oil: Provides anti-inflammatory and healing characteristics, making it perfect for soothing and repairing injured skin, including minor wounds and irritations.

5. Ginger Infused Castor Oil

Ingredients:

- *2 teaspoons dried ginger root or 1 tablespoon fresh ginger*
- *1 cup castor oil*

Instructions:

1. Combine dried or fresh ginger with castor oil in a sterile jar.
2. Infuse for 2-4 weeks using the cold or heated technique.
3. Strain and store in a dark bottle.

Benefits:

Ginger Essential Oil: Known for its warming and invigorating effects. Ginger-infused castor oil can help with muscle aches, improve circulation, and offer a warming effect.

Uses of Infused Castor Oil

1. Skin Care

Daily Moisturizer: Use infused castor oil to moisturize and soothe the skin. It can aid with dry spots, minor irritations, and overall skin health.

Anti-Inflammatory Treatment: Apply to areas of redness or inflammation to reduce swelling and promote healing.

2. Hair Care

Scalp Treatment: Massage into the scalp to promote hair growth and improve scalp health.

Conditioning: Use as a deep conditioning treatment to boost hair hydration and luster.

3. Nail and Cuticle Care

Strengthening: Apply to nails and cuticles to strengthen and hydrate.

Repairing: Helps with brittle nails and dry cuticles, promoting overall nail health.

1. Hibiscus Infused Castor Oil

Ingredients:

- *2 teaspoons dried hibiscus flowers*
- *1 cup castor oil*

Instructions:

1. Combine the dried hibiscus flowers and castor oil in a sterilized glass container.
2. Infuse using the cold or warm approach for 2-4 weeks.
3. Filter and keep in a bottle made of dark glass.

Benefits:

Hibiscus Essential Oil: Rich in antioxidants and vitamins A and C, hibiscus-infused castor oil helps to brighten the skin, even out skin tone, and minimize the appearance of dark spots. It also supports hair health by giving moisture and strength, making it particularly good for dry or damaged hair.

2. Nettle Infused Castor Oil

Ingredients:

- *2 teaspoons dried nettle leaves*
- *1 cup castor oil*

Instructions:

1. Combine dried nettle leaves and castor oil in a sterilized jar.
2. Infuse for 2-4 weeks using the cold or heated technique.
3. Filter and keep in a bottle made of dark glass.

Benefits:

Nettle Essential Oil: Known for its rich mineral content, including iron and vitamins A and C. Nettle-infused castor oil is ideal for encouraging hair growth, enhancing scalp health, and addressing issues such as dandruff and hair thinning. It also has anti-inflammatory qualities that can aid skin health.

3. Jasmine Infused Castor Oil

Ingredients:

- *2 teaspoons dried jasmine flowers*
- *1 cup castor oil*

Instructions:

1. Combine dried jasmine blossoms and castor oil in a sterilized jar.
2. Infuse for 2-4 weeks using the cold or heated technique.
3. Filter and keep in a bottle made of dark glass.

Benefits:

Jasmine Essential Oil: Provides a calming and uplifting smell while giving hydrating and anti-aging properties. Jasmine-infused castor oil is ideal for moisturizing dry skin, enhancing skin elasticity, and creating a beautiful complexion. It also aids in stress relief and relaxation.

4. Clove Infused Castor Oil

Ingredients:

- *2 teaspoons whole cloves*
- *1 cup castor oil*

Instructions:

1. Combine whole cloves and castor oil in a sterilized jar.

2. Infuse for 2-4 weeks using the cold or heated technique.
3. Filter and keep in a bottle made of dark glass.

Benefits:

Clove Essential Oil: Known for its antibacterial and anti-inflammatory qualities. Clove-infused castor oil is useful in boosting skin healing and treating acne-causing germs. It can also be used to ease muscle pains and joint pain because of its warming and relaxing qualities.

5. Thyme Infused Castor Oil

Ingredients:

- *2 teaspoons dried thyme leaves*
- *1 cup castor oil*

Instructions:

1. Combine dried thyme leaves and castor oil in a sterilized jar.
2. Infuse for 2-4 weeks using the cold or heated technique.
3. Filter and keep in a bottle made of dark glass.

Benefits:

Thyme Essential Oil: Known for its antibacterial and antifungal qualities. Thyme-infused castor oil is useful for treating scalp disorders such as dandruff and fungal infections. It also enhances general scalp health and can help with hair growth. For skincare, it helps to detoxify and cure the skin.

Precautions

Allergic Reactions: Perform a patch test before usage to ensure you do not have an allergic reaction to the infused oil.

Quality of Ingredients: Use high-quality, organic ingredients to achieve the greatest outcomes and avoid contamination.

Storage: Store infused oils in a dark, cold place to prevent oxidation and improve shelf life.

Precautions and Side Effects of Castor Oil

1. Potential Allergic Reactions

Understanding Allergic Reactions:

Symptoms: Allergic reactions to castor oil are relatively infrequent but can occur. Symptoms may include redness, irritation, swelling, or a rash at the site of application. In severe situations, symptoms could extend to hives, trouble breathing, or anaphylactic reactions.

Patch Test: Before using castor oil extensively, it's advised to perform a patch test.

Apply a small amount of the oil to a discreet area of the skin, such as the inner forearm, and wait 24 hours to detect any adverse effects. If you notice redness, irritation, or swelling, discontinue use and consult a healthcare provider.

How to Manage Allergic Reactions:

Discontinue Use: If you observe any signs of an allergic response after taking castor oil, discontinue using it immediately.

Clean the Area: Wash the affected area with gentle soap and water to remove any remaining oil.

Seek Medical Attention: For severe reactions, such as difficulty breathing or substantial swelling, seek emergency medical treatment immediately. For milder symptoms, consult a healthcare provider for advice on therapy.

2. Safe Usage Guidelines

General Recommendations:

Use in Moderation: While castor oil has many benefits, it should be used in moderation. Excessive application can lead to irritation or other negative effects.

Avoid Sensitive places: Be cautious when using castor oil in sensitive places, such as the eyes, mucous membranes, or broken skin. To avoid causing irritation, it is best to avoid applying in certain areas.

Follow guidelines: Adhere to the specified dosages and guidelines for internal ingestion or exterior application. Overuse might lead to harmful effects.

Quality of Oil: Ensure you are using high-quality, pure castor oil, ideally cold-pressed and organic, to eliminate potential impurities and additions that could irritate.

For Specific Uses:

Internal Use: If using castor oil internally (e.g., for constipation), start with a minimal dose and follow the prescribed guidelines. Excessive consumption might lead to gastrointestinal disorders such as diarrhea or cramps.

Topical Application: For skin and hair treatments, limit the frequency of application to avoid overloading the skin or scalp with oil. Two to three times a week is usually plenty.

3. When to Consult a Doctor

Consulting a Doctor:

Persistent Irritation: If you feel persistent skin irritation or other unpleasant consequences after taking castor oil, visit a healthcare expert. Persistent inflammation may require medical treatment or a new approach to skincare.

Allergic Reactions: If you suspect an allergic reaction, especially if it involves severe symptoms such as trouble breathing, swelling, or hives, get medical treatment immediately.

Internal Use Issues: If you have severe stomach discomfort, lengthy diarrhea, or other strange symptoms after taking castor oil, visit a healthcare provider. They can provide information on safe use and treat any potential underlying concerns.

Pre-existing disorders: If you have pre-existing health disorders, especially those affecting the digestive system, skin, or immune system, check with with your doctor before using castor oil. They can assist assess if castor oil is acceptable for you and advise on safe consumption.

Pregnancy and Breastfeeding:

Consult Your Doctor: Pregnant or breastfeeding individuals should consult a healthcare provider before using castor oil. While castor oil is widely used in labor induction, its safety for other purposes during pregnancy and breastfeeding should be examined by a medical expert.

Interactions with Medications:

Drug Interactions: If you are taking drugs or undergoing medical procedures, ask your healthcare professional before using castor oil. It's crucial to check there are no conflicts between castor oil and your medications.

Always prioritize your safety and consult healthcare specialists as needed to ensure that castor oil is utilized successfully and appropriately for your unique needs

Chapter Nine

Frequently Asked Questions (FAQs)

100 frequently asked questions (FAQs) about castor oil, covering its uses, benefits, and practical considerations:

1. What is castor oil?

Castor oil is a vegetable oil that is extracted from the seeds of the Ricinus communis plant. Due to its distinctive composition of fatty acids, particularly ricinoleic acid, it is recognized for its diverse therapeutic and cosmetic application.

2. How is castor oil made?

Castor oil is derived from castor beans by either cold pressing or expeller pressing techniques. The beans are crushed and the oil is extracted from the residue.

3. What are the basic components of castor oil?

Castor oil is mostly constituted of ricinoleic acid, a monounsaturated fatty acid, along with other fatty acids such as oleic and linoleic acids.

4. How may castor oil aid hair growth?

Castor oil stimulates hair growth by increasing blood circulation to the scalp and delivering necessary nutrients. Its ricinoleic acid helps to balance scalp pH and minimize irritation.

5. Is castor oil good for acne treatment?

Yes, castor oil has antibacterial and anti-inflammatory qualities that can help reduce acne. It is beneficial for relieving irritation and cleansing the top layer of skin.

6. Can castor oil be used for treating constipation?

Castor oil serves as a stimulating laxative and can help relieve constipation. It works by stimulating the intestines to encourage bowel motions.

7. How should castor oil be applied to the skin?

Castor oil can be applied directly to the the outermost skin or combined with other oils. It is preferable to apply it in small quantities and massage it into the desired location.

8. Can castor oil be used on sensitive skin?

Castor oil is generally safe for sensitive skin, however, it's important to run a patch test first to verify there is no adverse reaction.

9. How often should castor oil be administered for hair growth?

Castor oil can be applied 1-2 times per week to promote hair growth. It is essential to maintain consistency in order to observe results.

10. Can castor oil assist with joint pain?

Yes, castor oil's anti-inflammatory qualities can help ease joint pain and muscular aches when used topically.

11. Is it safe to swallow castor oil?

Castor oil can be consumed in tiny quantities as a laxative, but it should be administered under medical supervision to minimize negative effects.

12. How do you preserve castor oil?

To prevent oxidation and extend the shelf life of castor oil, it should be stored in a tightly sealed container in a cold, dark location.

13. Can castor oil be taken during pregnancy?

Castor oil is sometimes used to induce labor, but it should only be administered under the advice of a healthcare expert during pregnancy.

14. Can castor oil be used on pets?

Castor oil should be used gently on dogs, and it's recommended to consult a veterinarian before applying it.

15. What are the differences between cold-pressed and expeller-pressed castor oil?

Cold-pressed castor oil is extracted without heat, conserving more nutrients, while expeller-pressed oil is extracted using heat, which can alter some qualities.

16. How do you make castor oil infusions?

To produce an infusion, blend castor oil with dried herbs or botanicals and allow it to steep for a few weeks. Strain and store the infused oil.

17. Can castor oil assist with dry scalp?

Yes, castor oil helps hydrate and soothe a dry scalp, reducing flakiness and promoting healthier hair growth.

18. How do you use castor oil for nail care?

Apply castor oil to your nails and cuticles to strengthen and moisturize them. Regular application can help prevent brittleness and dryness.

19. Can castor oil be used for anti-aging?

Castor oil's hydrating and antioxidant characteristics can help minimize the appearance of fine lines and wrinkles, making it effective for anti-aging.

20. How do you apply castor oil for an eyelash boost?

Apply a small amount of castor oil to the base of your eyelashes before bedtime using a clean brush or applicator.

21. Can castor oil be used for sunburn?

Castor oil can help soothe and hydrate burnt skin, aiding healing and minimizing discomfort.

22. How does castor oil assist with dandruff?

Castor oil's antifungal and hydrating qualities can help eliminate dandruff by addressing dry scalp and fungal infections.

23. Is castor oil effective for curing stretch marks?

Castor oil can help improve the look of stretch marks by hydrating the skin and boosting collagen production.

24. How can you remove castor oil from the hair?

Castor oil can be removed with a clarifying shampoo or a mixture of baking soda and water to ensure all residues are washed out.

25. Can castor oil be used for diaper rash?

Yes, castor oil can be used to relieve and treat diaper rash due to its anti-inflammatory and moisturizing characteristics.

26. What is the shelf life of castor oil?

Castor oil normally has a shelf life of 1-2 years when stored correctly in a cold, dark environment.

27. How do you perform a patch test with castor oil?

Apply a small amount of castor oil to a small area of the skin and wait 24 hours to check for any signs of irritation or allergic response.

28. Can castor oil be used in cooking?

Castor oil is not suggested for cooking or ingestion due to its severe laxative effect and probable toxicity in large quantities.

29. How do you use castor oil for a face mask?

Mix castor oil with other natural substances like honey or yogurt, apply on the face, let for 15-20 minutes, and then rinse off.

30. Is castor oil suitable for all hair types?

Castor oil is generally acceptable for all hair types, although individuals with fine hair should use it sparingly to avoid weighing it down.

31. Can castor oil be used to remove makeup?

Castor oil can be used as a gentle makeup remover, especially for waterproof makeup, by kneading it onto the skin and then wiping it off with a cloth.

32. How may castor oil be used in a bath?

Add a few tablespoons of castor oil to a warm bath to help hydrate and soothe the skin.

33. Can castor oil be used for ear infections?

Castor oil should not be used to treat ear infections without medical supervision. It is recommended to visit a healthcare expert for suitable treatment.

34. How do you use castor oil for foot care?

Apply castor oil to your feet, especially the heels and cuticles, to hydrate and soften. Consider using it as part of a relaxing foot soak.

35. Is it possible to use castor oil as a carrier oil for essential oils?

Yes, castor oil can be used as a carrier oil to dilute essential oils for safe topical administration.

36. How does castor oil help with minor wounds?

Castor oil's antibacterial and moisturizing properties promote the healing process and prevent infection in minor wounds.

37. Can castor oil be used for hemorrhoids?

Castor oil can provide relief from hemorrhoid discomfort due to its anti-inflammatory effects, but it should be used with caution and under medical counsel.

38. What is the process for creating a castor oil compress?

Soak a cloth in castor oil, apply it to the afflicted region, and cover it with a plastic wrap or towel. Leave on for thirty to sixty minutes before removing.

39. Can castor oil be used to treat warts?

Castor oil's antiviral characteristics can assist with warts, but treatment should be consistent, and it's important to see a healthcare expert.

40. How may castor oil be used for sun protection?

Castor oil does not provide sun protection. Use sunscreen for protection against UV rays and castor oil for hydrating post-sun exposure.

41. Can castor oil be used for decreasing cellulite?

Castor oil's hydrating and anti-inflammatory qualities may help improve the appearance of cellulite when taken frequently.

42. Is castor oil effective for bruises?

Castor oil can aid in healing bruises by improving circulation and lowering inflammation, but it is not a substitute for medical therapy.

43. How may castor oil be used in aromatherapy?

Castor oil can be combined with essential oils to produce bespoke aromatherapy blends for relaxation, stress alleviation, or other therapeutic applications.

44. Can castor oil be used for colds or coughs?

Castor oil is not a primary treatment for colds or coughs. Consult a healthcare provider for proper remedies and treatments.

45. How can castor oil help with menstruation cramps?

Castor oil can be used in a warm compress to treat menstrual cramps by lowering muscle tension and inflammation.

46. Can castor oil be used for teeth whitening?

Castor oil is not typically used for tooth whitening. For oral health, it's better to utilize solutions specifically intended for tooth whitening.

47. How do you produce a castor oil and essential oil blend?

Combine castor oil with a few drops of your choice essential oil in a glass bottle. Shake thoroughly and use as needed for topical application or aromatherapy.

48. Is castor oil safe for children?

Castor oil can be used for children, but it should be used carefully and under the advice of a healthcare expert, especially for internal usage.

49. How can you use castor oil to prevent split ends?

Apply a small amount of castor oil to the ends of your hair to prevent split ends and add moisture and protection.

50. Can castor oil be used for arthritis?

Castor oil's anti-inflammatory qualities may provide relief from arthritis symptoms when used as a heated compress. Consult a healthcare provider for complete arthritis management.

51. Can castor oil be used to brighten dark spots?

Yes, castor oil's hydrating and regenerative characteristics can help lessen the appearance of black spots and even out skin tone over time.

52. How does castor oil assist with chapped lips?

Castor oil provides deep hydration and develops a protective barrier, making it beneficial for healing and preventing chapped lips.

53. Is it possible to treat cold sores with castor oil?

Castor oil may help ease the agony of cold sores due to its anti-inflammatory characteristics, but it should not replace antiviral medications.

54. How do you use castor oil for a face massage?

Apply a tiny amount of castor oil to your face and gently massage in circular motions to promote relaxation and boost skin moisture.

55. Is castor oil effective for curing eczema?

Castor oil's moisturizing and anti-inflammatory characteristics can help ease eczema symptoms, but it should be taken as part of a full treatment approach.

56. How can castor oil be used for under-eye circles?

Gently apply a tiny amount of castor oil beneath the eyes before bed to help moisturize and decrease the look of dark circles.

57. Is it possible to treat fungal infections using castor oil?

Castor oil has antifungal characteristics that can aid in treating small fungal infections, but it's vital to visit a healthcare expert for severe cases.

58. How does castor oil assist with hair loss?

Castor oil promotes hair development by increasing circulation to the scalp, decreasing inflammation, and delivering necessary nutrients.

59. Can castor oil be used for sunburn relief?

Yes, castor oil can soothe damaged skin by providing moisture and lowering irritation, but it's best used in conjunction with other sunburn remedies.

60. How do you prepare a castor oil bath soak?

Add a few tablespoons of castor oil to a warm bath to help hydrate and relax your body. Mix well to achieve even distribution.

61. Can castor oil assist with menstrual irregularities?

Castor oil is traditionally used to induce labor and regulate menstrual flow, but any use for menstrual abnormalities should be reviewed with a healthcare expert.

62. How can castor oil be used for a scalp treatment?

Apply castor oil directly to the scalp and massage in. After leaving it on for thirty to sixty minutes, use shampoo to remove it.

63. Can castor oil be used for eliminating warts?

Castor oil's antiviral qualities may help in treating warts, however, persistent warts should be checked and treated by a healthcare expert.

64. How does castor oil help with muscle soreness?

Castor oil can be used in a warm compress to reduce muscle discomfort by improving circulation and lowering inflammation.

65. Can castor oil be used for scar healing?

Yes, castor oil can aid in minimizing the appearance of scars by hydrating and encouraging skin regeneration.

66. How do you prepare a castor oil foot soak?

Add 2-3 teaspoons of castor oil to a basin of warm water. Soak your feet for 20-30 minutes to soften and hydrate.

67. Can castor oil be used for postpartum care?

Castor oil can be used in postpartum care for its relaxing and healing effects, but contact a healthcare expert for specific suggestions.

68. How may castor oil be used for relaxation?

Use castor oil in a warm compress or add it to a bath to encourage relaxation and ease stress.

69. Can castor oil help with psoriasis?

Castor oil's moisturizing and anti-inflammatory effects can help manage psoriasis symptoms, but it should be used alongside other therapies prescribed by a healthcare expert.

70. How do you use castor oil for a thorough conditioning treatment?

Apply castor oil to damp hair after combining it with other conditioning products. Let it sit for half an hour or more, then rinse with shampoo.

71. Can castor oil be used for earaches?

Castor oil should not be used for earaches without medical advice. It's best to visit a healthcare expert for effective therapy.

72. How can castor oil be used for treating dandruff?

Lightly massage the scalp with castor oil. To help reduce dandruff, let it on for a minimum of thirty minutes before washing it off.

73. Can castor oil assist with varicose veins?

Castor oil can help alleviate the irritation of varicose veins, but it should be used in conjunction with other medical therapies and lifestyle changes.

74. How do you use castor oil for a relaxing skin treatment?

Apply castor oil directly to sore or inflamed skin regions to provide calming treatment and encourage healing.

75. Can castor oil be used for treating burns?

Castor oil can be used to treat mild burns and promote healing, but serious burns require emergency medical assistance.

76. How can castor oil help with indigestion?

Castor oil is occasionally used to alleviate indigestion by accelerating digestion and increasing bowel movements.

77. Can castor oil be used for treating athlete's foot?

Castor oil's antifungal characteristics may assist with athlete's foot, but it's best taken alongside other antifungal therapies.

78. How may castor oil be utilized in homemade skincare products?

Castor oil can be included in DIY skincare products like lotions, balms, and masks to boost their moisturizing and healing characteristics.

79. Can castor oil assist with weary eyes?

Castor oil can help ease weary eyes when applied around the eye area to alleviate dryness and enhance moisture.

80. How do you use castor oil for a DIY face serum?

Combine castor oil with different carrier oils and essential oils to create a bespoke face serum. Every day, apply a few drops on your face.

81. Can castor oil be used for oral health?

Castor oil is not commonly utilized for oral health. For oral care, utilize items specifically intended for dental hygiene.

82. How does castor oil help with muscle cramps?

Castor oil's anti-inflammatory characteristics can help relax muscles and relieve the pain associated with cramps when used in a warm compress.

83. Can castor oil be used for curing shingles?

Castor oil may provide calming relief for shingles-related discomfort, but it should not substitute medical treatment.

84. How can you use castor oil for a soothing lip balm?

Mix castor oil with beeswax and other hydrating oils to produce a pleasant lip balm. Apply as needed to keep lips moisturized.

85. Can castor oil be useful for treating cold or flu symptoms?

Castor oil is not a major treatment for cold or flu symptoms. Use it for supportive care like calming muscles or skin, and see a healthcare expert for particular treatments.

86. How may castor oil be used for muscle relaxation?

Apply castor oil as a warm compress to tight muscles to help relax and reduce tension.

87. Can castor oil be used for relaxation and sleep?

Castor oil can be used in a bath or as a massage oil to promote relaxation and improve sleep quality.

88. How does castor oil assist with age spots?

Castor oil's hydrating characteristics can help minimize the appearance of age spots by encouraging skin regeneration and smoothing out skin tone.

89. Is it possible to treat insect bites using castor oil?

Castor oil's anti-inflammatory and calming characteristics can help lessen the agony and minimize swelling from insect bites.

90. How do you make a castor oil and essential oil blend for sleep?

Combine castor oil with essential oils like lavender or chamomile in a glass bottle. Use the blend in a diffuser or apply it to pulse points before bedtime.

91. Can castor oil assist with toothaches?

Castor oil is not a standard therapy for toothaches. Consult a dentist for proper examination and treatment.

92. How do you use castor oil for an eye mask?

Combine castor oil with other nutritious oils and apply it to the under-eye area. Let it sit for ten to fifteen minutes before removing.

93. Can castor oil be used for treating hair lice?

Castor oil may help treat hair lice by smothering the lice, but it should be used with other lice treatments for success.

94. How does castor oil assist general skin health?

Castor oil hydrates, calms, and stimulates skin healing, making it excellent for keeping healthy and hydrated skin.

95. Can castor oil be used for treating sinus congestion?

Castor oil is not commonly used for sinus congestion. Consult a healthcare provider for proper treatments for sinus difficulties.

96. How do you use castor oil for a body scrub?

Mix castor oil with sugar or salt to create a natural exfoliating body scrub. Massage onto the skin in circular strokes and rinse.

97. Can castor oil be used to enhance circulation?

Castor oil's warming action can aid improve circulation when used in a massage or heated compress.

98. How can castor oil assist with cracked heels?

Castor oil's hydrating qualities might help heal and soothe damaged heels when used consistently.

99. Can castor oil be used for treating nausea?

Castor oil is not often used for nausea. Consult a healthcare provider for recommended solutions for nausea.

100. How do you use castor oil for a pleasant foot massage?

Mix castor oil with a few drops of essential oil and use it to massage your feet, focusing on any areas of tension or stiffness.

www.ingramcontent.com/pod-product-compliance
Lightning Source LLC
Chambersburg PA
CBHW081807250726
48653CB00010B/3825